Exercise and Wellness for Older Adults

Practical Programming Strategies

SECOND EDITION

Exercise and Wellness for Older Adults

Practical Programming Strategies

SECOND EDITION

Kay A. Van Norman, MS

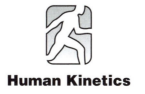

Human Kinetics

Library of Congress Cataloging-in-Publication Data

Van Norman, Kay A., 1957-
  Exercise and wellness for older adults : practical programming strategies / Kay A. Van Norman. -- 2nd ed.
    p. ; cm.
  Rev. ed. of: Exercise programming for older adults / Kay A. Van Norman. c1995.
  Includes bibliographical references and index.
  ISBN-13: 978-0-7360-5768-4 (soft cover)
  ISBN-10: 0-7360-5768-4 (soft cover)
  1. Exercise for older people. 2. Physical fitness for older people. I. Van Norman, Kay A., 1957- Exercise programming for older adults. II. Title.
  [DNLM: 1. Exercise. 2. Physical Fitness. 3. Aged. 4. Aging. 5. Health Promotion. 6. Holistic Health. QT 255 V217e 2010]
  GV482.6.V36 2010
  613.7'0446--dc22
                                    2009048063
ISBN-10: 0-7360-5768-4 (print)
ISBN-13: 978-0-7360-5768-4 (print)

This book is a revised edition of *Exercise Programming for Older Adults,* published in 1995 by Human Kinetics, Inc.

The Web addresses cited in this text were current as of January, 2010, unless otherwise noted.

Acquisitions Editor: Judy Patterson Wright, PhD; **Developmental Editors:** Jillian Evans and Kevin Matz; **Assistant Editors:** Casey A. Gentis and Steven Calderwood; **Copyeditor:** Julie Anderson; **Indexer:** Betty Frizzéll; **Permission Manager:** Dalene Reeder; **Graphic Designer:** Dawn Sills; **Graphic Artist:** Dawn Sills; **Cover Designer:** Bob Reuther; **Photographer (cover):** © Friedrich Stark/Imago/Icon SMI; **Photographer (interior):** © Human Kinetics, unless otherwise noted. Photos on pp. 116, 123-126, 128-131, 133-136 courtesy of Casey Lipok Photography; photo on p. 153 Bill Crump/Brand X Pictures; **Photo Asset Manager:** Laura Fitch; **Visual Production Assistant:** Joyce Brumfield; **Photo Production Manager:** Jason Allen; **Art Manager:** Kelly Hendren; **Associate Art Manager:** Alan L. Wilborn; **Illustrator:** Keri Evans; **Printer:** Versa Press

We thank Clark-Lindsey Village in Urbana, Illinois, for assistance in providing the location for the photo shoot for this book.

Printed in the United States of America   10 9 8 7 6 5 4 3 2 1

The paper in this book is certified under a sustainable forestry program.

Human Kinetics
Web site: www.HumanKinetics.com

United States: Human Kinetics
P.O. Box 5076
Champaign, IL 61825-5076
800-747-4457
e-mail: humank@hkusa.com

Canada: Human Kinetics
475 Devonshire Road Unit 100
Windsor, ON N8Y 2L5
800-465-7301 (in Canada only)
e-mail: info@hkcanada.com

Europe: Human Kinetics
107 Bradford Road
Stanningley
Leeds LS28 6AT, United Kingdom
+44 (0) 113 255 5665
e-mail: hk@hkeurope.com

Australia: Human Kinetics
57A Price Avenue
Lower Mitcham, South Australia 5062
08 8372 0999
e-mail: info@hkaustralia.com

New Zealand: Human Kinetics
P.O. Box 80
Torrens Park, South Australia 5062
0800 222 062
e-mail: info@hknewzealand.com

E3367

Contents

Preface

Since writing *Exercise Programming for Older Adults* in 1995, I've experienced a dramatic paradigm shift. I used to focus on programming to meet the needs of adults over 55 but now realize that age has very little to do with functional ability and even less to do with what a person is capable of than almost any other factor. I know that expectations, personal beliefs, and intent affect outcomes, regardless of age. For example, many people with physical disabilities accomplish amazing things, like the blind man who climbed Mount Everest and the thousands of disabled athletes who compete in Paralympics. Research clearly demonstrates the ability of the human body to retain high levels of function through the life span (Spirduso et al., 2005). One need only observe the rapidly growing number of Senior Olympians running, jumping, and powerlifting against stiff competition or read longitudinal studies done around the world showing people who are 90 years old and older actively engaged in physically challenging lifestyles to see the possibilities for lifelong health and vitality (Buettner, 2005).

I have changed my programming approach from an age-based perspective to one based on function. Programming for older adults as we know it in the industry today could well be named programming for adults who have been sedentary or have functional limitations and so require specialized programming. Don't discount the importance of this difference in perspective, because one of the biggest challenges for wellness specialists is to convince adults of all ages that although decline in some physical parameters with age is predictable, functional dependence is not inevitable.

A severe physical disability or functional challenge does not necessarily define what a person is capable of accomplishing. For example, Kyle Maynard became a successful high school varsity wrestler despite being born with arms ending at the elbows and legs ending at the knees (Maynard, 2005), demonstrating the power of elements like personal beliefs, expectations, and intent to influence behaviors and outcomes. Chapter 3, Psychosocial Aspects of Programming, examines how these often-overlooked elements affect behavior and offers insight on how to engage them in a positive manner to improve well-being.

Professionals in wellness promotion must lead the way by changing our mind-set, our language, and our approach to programming. We must incorporate strategies to overcome psychosocial barriers to healthy lifestyle habits and offer programming to maximize functional ability regardless of age or physical challenge. We must also embrace the relationship between the body, mind, and spirit that support well-being.

This book will help wellness professionals make the paradigm shift from expectations of decline to an age-neutral focus on maximizing functional ability. The book provides specialized programming for adults who have diminished physical function or special conditions requiring modified programs. It also supports the shift from a fitness focus to a whole-person wellness focus that fully engages individuals as full partners in well-being, rather than customers of wellness strategies.

Like the first edition, this book provides an overview of the field of adult wellness, including a synopsis of population demographics and a review of challenges and opportunities in the wellness industry (chapter 1). It also discusses the shift from a fitness to a wellness focus in health promotion programs. It offers a brief overview of the functioning of the cardiopulmonary, musculoskeletal, and nervous systems; changes common with inactivity and aging; and special conditions that affect exercise safety (chapter 2). The book provides program guidelines and specific programming for both land- and water-based exercise (chapters 4-6) and concludes with strategies to develop and promote your wellness program in community-based as well as senior living environments (chapter 7).

The new elements of this edition include the following:

- A complete chapter on the psychosocial components of aging and wellness
- Introduction of the whole-person wellness concept and strategies to integrate the six dimensions of wellness into programming

- Strength and power training protocols and specific programming
- Material on the unique challenges and opportunities in senior living environments plus programming approaches for this venue

This edition has been much more difficult to write than the first one. Before, it was pretty convenient to make broad statements like "older adults need _____." I'm somewhat embarrassed now that I even wrote those statements, so I've worked hard to avoid those types of generalizations. I've also tried to strike a balance between using an age-neutral focus and providing the information necessary to create programs for people who have functional deficits. It's a balancing act and I have been as consistent as possible. I wish you the best of luck in your programs and thank you for your commitment to this field. Let's all keep it moving forward!

Acknowledgments

I first thank my husband, George Gebhardt, and sons, Brock and Cole. Once again you've had to put up with piles of papers on the dining room table and my attention directed at the computer for hours on end. I appreciate your love and support. I also thank my personal cheerleaders Chris Van Burgh and Lois Syth, who kept me moving forward on this project at times when I was stalled.

Thanks also go to all the models in the book who gave of their time so freely and to Clark Lindsey Village in Urbana, Illinois, where many photos were taken. Special thanks go to my friends and horseback riding buddies, who demonstrate by example how to stay active, live fully, and age well. Bob Jordan, Eldo Heinle, Kay Moore, Mary Jane Johnson, and Grace France—thanks for blazing the trail. I look forward to riding the mountains with you for many more years to come.

I thank the many colleagues I've worked with and learned from over the years in the Council on Aging and Adult Development, National Council on Aging, Keiser Institute on Aging, and International Council on Active Aging. Finally, to Jan Montague, my friend and colleague—thanks for opening the door to whole-person wellness and providing many years of insight, collaboration, and friendship.

Aging and Wellness

It is an exciting time to be involved in exercise and wellness programming for older adults, which is the fastest-growing market in the health promotion industry. More people than ever before recognize the importance and the *possibility* of retaining vitality through the life span. Health promotion and senior service organizations are working hard to educate adults about the benefits of a healthy, active lifestyle, and there are more opportunities than ever to engage in healthy lifestyle programs. The aging of the baby boomer generation has resulted in a dramatic increase in the numbers of adults older than 65. Federal agencies, driven by these changes in age demographics, are seeking practical strategies to keep people well in body, mind, and spirit throughout the life span.

Health promotion is evolving from disease prevention and management, which is termed the *medical model* and has focused on health screenings and exercise programs, into a whole-person wellness model recognizing the importance of body, mind, and spirit in overall well-being. Research proving the health benefits of regular exercise is joined by studies showing the importance of engaging the mind and emotions in prevention and healing (Cohen, 2005; Ray, 2004). The demand for programs that effectively engage the whole person— body, mind, and spirit—on the path to well-being will significantly affect the health promotion and wellness industry and offers many opportunities for professionals ready to make the shift from an age-based fitness focus to a function-based wellness focus.

The aging of baby boomers provides an excellent opportunity to make a radical shift in perceptions and approaches. This group as a whole is less inclined than past generations to accept limitations imposed by ageist stereotypes. Many mature adults reject the expectation of deteriorating health and actively seek positive alternatives. Elite athletes like Lance Armstrong and Olympic athletes age 40 and older push themselves to higher levels of performance, shattering the myth that physical potential peaks around age 30. Many nonathletes are also aging with amazing vitality and demonstrating that simply staying fully engaged in life offers the opportunity for vitality, meaning, purpose, and quality of life throughout the life span. I look forward to a time when the majority of adults believe not just in the *possibility* of aging well but also in the *probability* of aging well.

This chapter provides a synopsis of age demographics around the world. It highlights how wellness programs can help adults remain healthy and engaged in life throughout their lives. The chapter identifies the five levels of physical function, which you can use to identify and meet the needs of adults at various levels of functional ability. The chapter also introduces the concept of whole-person wellness and outlines its six main components: physical, social, emotional, spiritual, intellectual, and vocational. Finally, this chapter discusses the industries and organizations related to senior wellness, including fitness, senior-living, community-based recreation, senior service, and health and aging organizations.

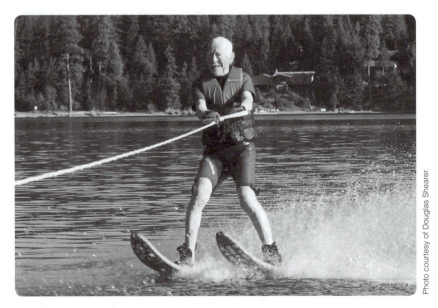

Age is just a number.

Photo courtesy of Douglas Shearer.

AGING WORLD POPULATIONS

At this writing, the world population of people 65 and older was 495 million. That number is projected to increase to 997 million by 2030. With 19.1% of Italy's population older than 65, Italy is listed as the world's "oldest" major country, with Japan a close second at 19%. The remaining top 20 of the world's oldest countries are all in Europe. The United States ranks 38th in the world, with 12.4% of its population age 65 and older (Kinsella and Phillips, 2005). Figure 1.1 illustrates how the populations of those aged 65 and older are projected to increase by 2050 in selected countries.

The majority of people aged 65 and older in industrialized nations do not engage in physical activity at the level necessary to receive health benefits. Among adults older than 65, only 16% to 27% of Americans and less than one third of Canadians are regularly active. Only 3.5% of older adults in Italy are regularly physically active and another 2.2% are occasionally physically active. Given health and disability statistics of adults older than 65, governments around the world are concerned about the impact of the projected age-wave. Without intervention, sedentary adults around the world are at risk of losing the ability to function independently, which would put a tremendous strain on health care systems and the ability of governments

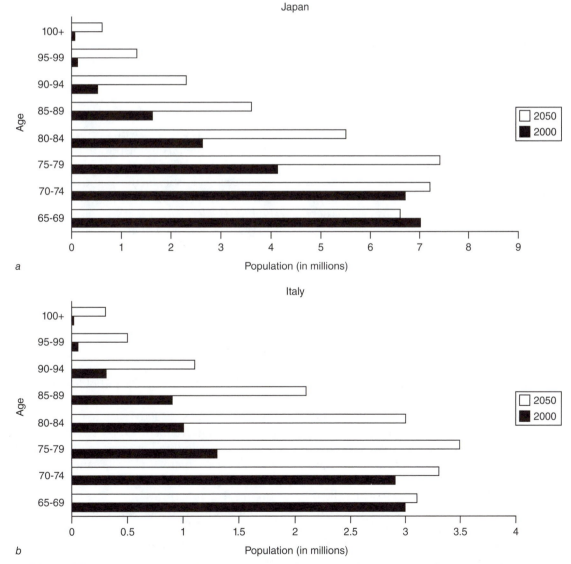

▶ **Figure 1.1** Populations aged 65 and older in *(a)* Japan, *(b)* Italy, and *(c)* Canada, both in the year 2000 and projected for 2050.

Data from U.S. Census Bureau, International Database.

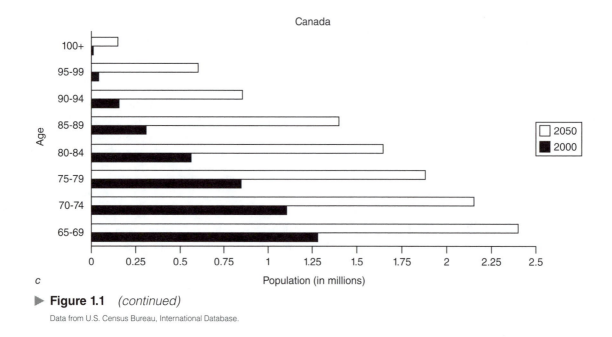

▶ **Figure 1.1** *(continued)*

Data from U.S. Census Bureau, International Database.

to care for large numbers of dependent people. For example, the World Health Organization (WHO) estimated that the total projected loss of income in China as a result of heart disease, stroke, and diabetes from 2005 to 2015 would be $558 billion in U.S. currency (WHO, 2005). Many countries are drafting national health policies to address the need to increase participation in physical activity and other healthy lifestyle programs (CDC, 2007; Benjamin et al., 2005; Lucidi et al., 2006; Rasinaho et al., 2007).

PROFILE OF OLDER AMERICANS

According to the U.S. Census Bureau, in 2004 there were 36.3 million people in America aged 65 and older, an increase of 3.1 million since 1994. Between 2004 and 2005, this age group increased by 457,000 people, accounting for 12% of the total population. The 65 and older population in the United States is projected to reach 86.7 million by 2050, making up 21% of the total population (see figure 1.2). Projections show that the U.S. population as a whole will increase by 49% from 2000 to 2050, while the 65 and older population will increase by an amazing 147% (Administration on Aging, 2005).

One of the fastest-growing segments of the older population is adults older than 85, who numbered 4.2 million in 2000 and are expected to reach 6.1 million by 2010 (a 40% increase in one decade) and

7.3 million by 2020 (a 44% increase in one decade). The number of centenarians (100 and older) in 2006 was estimated at 79,682, with a projected increase to 580,605 by 2040 (Administration on Aging, 2005). The AARP Web site (www.aarp.org) is an excellent resource for statistics on the 65 and older population and their lifestyle. Look for the regularly updated *Profiles of Older Americans* at www.aarp.org/research/surveys/stats/demo/agingtrends/articles/aresearch-import-519.html.

Health in an Aging America

Population demographics will drive continued growth in the senior wellness industry. Properly designed wellness programs can help older Americans retain functional independence and quality of life. In 2004, only 27% of persons aged 65 to 74 and 16% of persons 75 and older reported that they engaged in regular leisure-time physical activity. Lack of physical activity contributes to many of the conditions frequently reported in adults age 65 and older, including hypertension (51%), arthritis (48%), heart disease (31%), cancer (21%), and diabetes (16%) (Administration on Aging, 2005). Figure 1.3 illustrates the increase in disability common with increased age. Without intervention, increased numbers of Americans older than 85 will mean increased disability and increased health care costs. Wellness programs for adults should focus on preventing disability by maximizing endurance, mobility, balance, and muscular strength and power.

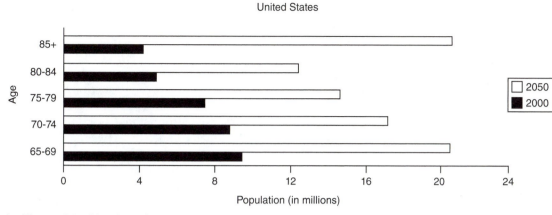

▶ **Figure 1.2** Number of people aged 65 and older in the United States, both in the year 2000 and projected for 2050.

Data from U.S. Census Bureau, International Database.

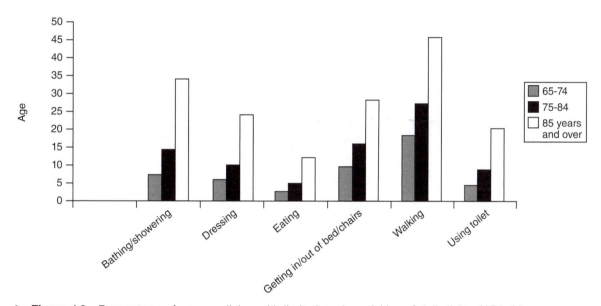

▶ **Figure 1.3** Percentage of persons living with limitations in activities of daily living (ADLs) by age group in 2003. Sample taken from noninstitutionalized adults older than 65.

U.S. Administration on Aging, 2008. Available: www.aoa.gov/AoARoot/Aging_Statistics/Profile/2008/16.aspx

Unhealthy lifestyles dramatically affect the health of children in America. Conditions such as diabetes and heart disease, long thought to be age related, are showing up in alarming numbers in sedentary children. The good news for all ages is that these conditions can be prevented or managed through positive lifestyle changes.

Maintaining Health Span and Productivity

For the past two decades, government and media outlets have predicted dire consequences resulting from aging world populations. However, the problems predicted to occur as a result of aging populations stem from advanced disability rather than just advanced age. They include the loss of health (i.e., a strain on health care systems); the loss of productivity (i.e., a diminished work force); and the loss of independence (i.e., a need for long-term care). If the number of people with unhealthy lifestyles (inactivity and poor nutrition) remains the same, a crisis will indeed accompany changing demographics. However, research proves that prevention works, and positive changes in the field of health and wellness promotion can help more adults than ever before embrace healthy lifestyles (CDC, 2007).

Regular exercise and other positive lifestyle choices help increase "health span," the length of time that a person can enjoy a healthy, active life. Improving the health span of adults can mitigate the presumed impact of aging demographics on the health care industry. There is less concern now than a decade ago about a diminished work force because many healthy adults of retirement age are opting to continue working in their professions or have found entirely new work interests. The predictions of tremendous economic strain on social programs have given way to a cautious optimism that this generation of retirees will volunteer many hours to help sustain social programs.

Maintaining Independence

Maintaining independence requires the ability to perform basic self-care. The standard definition of functional independence is that a person must be able to perform the basic activities of daily living (BADLs), including bathing, dressing, transferring (getting in and out of beds and chairs), walking, eating, and using the toilet, without assistance (Spirduso et al., 2005). Figure 1.3 (p. 5) illustrates the loss of functional independence common in people 85 years and older. Exercise, especially power training, has been proven to increase people's ability to perform ADLs.

Almost every functional task listed in figure 1.3 requires power to perform effectively, so anyone interested in improving the functional status of older adults must understand the difference between strength and power. Simply put, strength is the ability to generate force, and power is the ability to generate force quickly. For example, stand up very slowly from a chair (4-6 counts), sit back down, and then stand up quickly. Slowly rising from a chair primarily uses strength alone and so is more difficult than rising quickly, which is the normal sit-to-stand functional pattern requiring power (i.e., strength × speed). For more than 20 years researchers and professionals have known that strength training can improve function, yet the idea that all older adults should strength train is just now starting to become a mainstream concept. Recent power-training research consistently demonstrates that power training affects functional status significantly more than does strength training alone; however, power has not yet been embraced by health and wellness promotion professionals and incorporated into exercise programs (Fielding et al., 2002; Hazell et al., 2007; Miszko et al., 2003).

Professionals must bring power training to the forefront of programming as soon as possible by making the transition from programming for strength alone to programming for power. In a rapidly aging world, we cannot afford to let power research languish for years as changes in protocols trickle down to practitioners and older adults. Discuss the role of power in function with colleagues and clients and follow new research on the topic. Request that professional organizations like the International Council on Active Aging, the National Council on Aging, and the American Society on Aging address the issue of power and functional independence at yearly conferences. Read Hazell and colleagues' (2007) review of studies investigating the effect of strength and power training on ADL performance. Figure 1.4 illustrates the differences in ADL performance reported in strength and power research. Refer to chapters 4 and 5 for more information and practical strategies for incorporating strength and power training into programs.

Improving functional status requires more than just creating the right programs—adults have to participate to benefit! Professionals must convince adults that although loss of functional independence is highly predictable, it is not inevitable. Changing perceptions of aging and physical activity is the first step to engaging people as partners in well-being. Furthermore, the disability movement demonstrates how people can live vital active lives with adaptive equipment and minimal assistance even with significant physical limitations. This could be viewed as a person's *physical competence*, regardless of abilities or disabilities. Programs must focus on improving people's functional ability and their ability to adapt to changing circumstances, regardless of age. See chapter 3 for a discussion of psychosocial elements that influence physical activity behavior, functional independence, and quality of life and chapter 4 for specific strategies to engage adults as partners in well-being.

ATTITUDES TOWARD AGING

There is an appalling persistence of aging stereotypes in the media and consistent, negative emphasis on the outward signs of aging, such as wrinkling of the skin and gray hair. Youth-oriented boomers who succumb to the notion that aging is bad do everything to defy the outward signs of aging, driving the multibillion-dollar anti-aging industry. Negative representations of older adults in both visual and print media would have us believe there is nothing positive about aging; however, research shows that the majority of adults are satisfied with their age (Administration on Aging, 2005). *Mature*

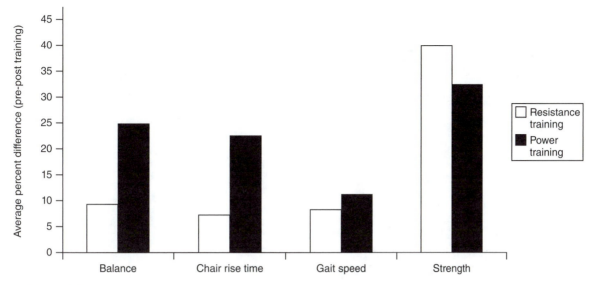

▶ **Figure 1.4** Differences in performance of activities of daily living resulting from strength versus power training.

Reprinted, by permission, from T. Hazell, K. Kenno, and J. Jakobi, 2007, "Functional benefit of power training for older adults," *Journal of Aging and Physical Activity* 15: 349-359.

Mind, The Positive Power of the Aging Brain (Cohen, 2005) is an excellent resource on positive aspects of aging. Dr. Cohen, a pioneer in the positive aging field, cites brain research showing how links develop between the right and left brain as a result of aging, improving many brain functions.

Most physical declines associated with aging result from inactivity and other poor lifestyle habits rather than just age (Spirduso et al., 2005). Other negative stereotypes like social isolation, decline of mental acuity, loss of status, and depression also result primarily from lifestyle habits, such as a lack of social, emotional, and intellectual engagement. Previous generations were led to believe that *age equals decline* and so more readily accepted the limitations imposed by overt ageism. The real shockwave to our youth-obsessed culture (and the businesses thriving on it) will be the growing movement of self-actualized boomers who reject the idea that aging itself is bad and instead redefine aging with an attitude of "yes, I'm 65, so what does that have to do with anything?"

Although many boomer-generation adults have different expectations of advanced age compared with previous generations, many are still affected by overt and subtle ageist attitudes and expectations, especially when faced with significant health challenges. Chapter 3 thoroughly discusses these expectations and offers strategies to overcome their impact. The timing is right to make a radical shift in perceptions of aging well, and the health promotion and wellness industry is in a perfect position to lead

the change. Group and individualized programs designed to address functional ability regardless of age will play a significant role in changing perceptions. Wellness specialists who help adults maximize function and capitalize on positive aspects of aging will be in high demand.

CHALLENGING BARRIERS AND CHANGING NEEDS

Exercise and wellness classes for adults must meet the needs of a diverse population: people who have been active throughout their lives and others who have been sedentary. Some adults will believe anything is possible with the right training, whereas others will believe that age limits their ability. Others will be affected by a condition requiring modified programs. The challenge for wellness specialists will be to safely meet the needs of participants without reinforcing the ageist stereotypes so common in our culture.

Fitness Needs

Fitness significantly influences the ability to maintain health and engage in work and recreational activities. Therefore, exercise programs should strive to enhance overall fitness, including cardiovascular endurance, flexibility, coordination, balance, agility, and muscular strength, power, and endurance. Age is a risk factor for conditions that

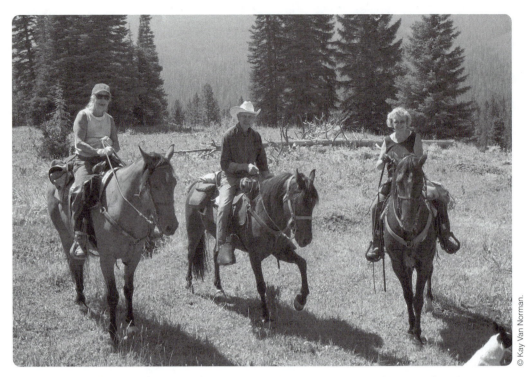

Grace France, Mary Jane Johnson, and Eldo Heinle, ages 66 to 80, enjoying the mountains of Montana.

significantly affect exercise safety, such as arthritis, osteoporosis, diabetes, joint and muscular dysfunction, and cardiovascular dysfunction. However, many of these conditions are now appearing in youth populations who demonstrate unhealthy lifestyles.

Regular exercise and proper nutrition offer significant protection from these and other chronic conditions. Wellness specialists must provide programming that addresses common conditions and risk factors without making assumptions based on age. The five levels of functional ability outlined next will help you program for needs rather than age.

In *Physical Dimensions of Aging* (2005), Spirduso identified five levels of functional ability: physically dependent, physically frail, physically independent, physically fit, and physically elite. Her definitions, outlined in table 1.1, provide a framework for identifying functional abilities of each level.

Physical levels of ability are also heavily influenced by attitudes and personal belief systems. Factors like self-concept and perception of abilities affect what a person is able to accomplish regardless of abilities or disabilities. Chapter 3 discusses these factors in detail. Refer to table 4.1 (p. 54) for a description of some basic needs common to each level of functional ability and strategies to help you identify and prioritize program goals to meet these needs.

Whole-Person Wellness

In the first edition of this book, I stated that social and emotional components of programming were more important in older adult classes than younger adult classes. I don't believe that anymore; rather, I think that the need for these components is entirely dependent on the person, regardless of age. Some people will seek out classes that actively facilitate social interaction; others will be satisfied with a program that sticks to the exercise and leaves interaction to chance. However, regardless of age, connection to a group improves exercise compliance. Classes should be actively structured to facilitate participant interaction and develop a sense of group cohesiveness. They must also be designed to engage multiple dimensions of health (body, mind, and spirit) on the path to wellness. See chapter 4 for specific strategies.

Wellness is defined by the National Wellness Institute (NWI) as optimal function in the physical, social, emotional, intellectual, spiritual, and vocational (or occupational) dimensions of health. Wellness is specific to a person's abilities and encompasses attitude, behavior, and personal

Table 1.1 Levels of Function

Category	Description
Physically dependent	People who cannot execute some or all of the basic activities of daily living, including dressing, bathing, transferring, toileting, feeding, and walking. These people are dependent on others for food and other basic functions of living.
Physically frail	People who can perform the basic activities of daily living but cannot perform some or all of the activities that are necessary to live independently, generally because of a debilitating disease or condition that physically challenges them daily.
Physically independent	People who live independently, usually without debilitating symptoms of major chronic diseases. However, many have low health and fitness reserves, placing them at risk for becoming physically frail after illness or injury.
Physically fit	People who exercise at least two times a week for their health, enjoyment, and well-being or engage regularly in a physically demanding job or hobby. Their health and fitness reserves put them at low risk for falling into the physically frail category.
Physically elite	People who train almost daily to either compete in sport tournaments or engage in a physically demanding job or recreational activity.

Based on W. Spirduso, 1995, *Physical Dimensions of Aging* (Champaign, IL: Human Kinetics).

beliefs (Montague and Van Norman, 1998). Jan Montague is widely credited with bringing the six-dimensional wellness model to the senior-living industry in the 1990s and has helped it become the gold standard of wellness programming for senior housing. Whole-person wellness is outlined in the widely used six-dimensional model seen on page 10.

The wellness model contrasts sharply with both the medical model, which defines health as the absence of disease, and the fitness model, which defines health as physical well-being. The medical model is largely reactive and problem focused, emphasizing assessments and treatment. The wellness model focuses on what is right with a person rather than what is wrong and encourages participation in activities to the best of one's ability. This model recognizes that the absence of disease alone does not make someone "well" and that many people with excellent physical fitness may have significant difficulties with other aspects of their lives. Conversely, some people with severe health conditions or significant physical challenges can demonstrate a high level of wellness.

The wellness approach calls for people to be active partners in their own well-being rather than customers of health services. The whole-person wellness wheel (figure 1.5), designed by Jan Montague, illustrates how each dimension of well-being is an important part of whole-person health. It also shows how each dimension is connected and interrelated. Finally, it demonstrates that personal wellness comes from the inside out and relies on elements like self-responsibility and self-efficacy to support well-being.

Understanding the six dimensions of wellness and their equal importance in supporting health can help you integrate multiple dimensions into your programming approaches. An exercise class addresses the physical dimension, of course, so start by adding at least one other dimension to a class. For example, to incorporate the emotional dimension into a physical exercise program, end the class with an uplifting quote or inspirational thought for the day. Encourage participants to bring their favorite quotations to class. Create opportunities for participants to interact socially during class: Add partner work, use social mixer dance routines, or arrange the class so participants stand in lines facing each other. Refer to chapter 5 for strategies for integrating multiple dimensions into programs. Also refer to chapter 3 for details on addressing attitudes, perceptions, and expectations that support self-responsibility for healthy aging.

The demand for programs that effectively address whole-person wellness will have a significant impact on the fitness, senior housing, and health promotion industries and will open many avenues of career growth for proactive professionals. Chapter 4 provides practical strategies to integrate whole-person wellness concepts into physical activity programs, and chapter 7 offers examples of how to use the wellness model as a framework for programming in senior-living environments.

WHOLE-PERSON WELLNESS OUTLINE

The six dimensions of the model are described here.

Physical Dimension

The physical dimension encourages participation in activities contributing to a high level of physical well-being, including physical activity, personal safety, medical self-care, and the appropriate use of the medical system. This dimension promotes increased knowledge about achieving healthy lifestyle habits and discourages negative, excessive behavior. The physical dimension includes these elements:

▶ Fitness

▶ Nutrition

▶ Weight management

▶ Functional abilities

▶ Healthy lifestyle habits

▶ Safety

▶ Health screenings

Social Dimension

The social dimension emphasizes the creation and maintenance of healthy relationships. It emphasizes interdependence with others and nature and encourages the pursuit of harmony within the family and community. The following actions fall into the social dimension:

▶ Respect oneself and others

▶ Respect differences

▶ Interact with others and the environment

▶ Create and maintain healthy relationships

▶ Enhance self-concept

Emotional Dimension

The emotional dimension emphasizes an awareness and acceptance of one's feelings. It reflects the degree to which a person feels positive and enthusiastic about herself and life. This dimension involves the capacity to accept oneself unconditionally, assess limitations and possibilities, develop autonomy, and cope with stress. The emotional dimension includes the following efforts:

▶ Express and recognize feelings

▶ Control stress

▶ Problem solve

▶ Manage success and failure

▶ Enhance self-esteem

▶ Identify personal expectations

Intellectual Dimension

The intellectual dimension promotes the use of the mind to create a greater understanding and appreciation of oneself, others, and the world. It involves the ability to think creatively and rationally and encourages people to expand knowledge and skills through a variety of resources and cultural activities. The following actions fall into the intellectual dimension:

- ▶ Engage in lifetime learning
- ▶ Actively use the mind
- ▶ Facilitate creative thinking
- ▶ Explore new ideas and interests

Spiritual Dimension

The spiritual dimension involves seeking meaning and purpose in life. It involves developing a strong sense of personal values and ethics and may or may not be religiously based. This dimension includes appreciation for the depth and expanse of life and natural forces that exist in the universe. It includes these components:

- ▶ Discovery of meaning and purpose in life
- ▶ Demonstration of values, morals, and ethics through behaviors
- ▶ Self-determination (not always religiously based)
- ▶ Feelings of love, hope, and abundance
- ▶ Reflection, contemplation, and meditation

Vocational Dimension

The vocational dimension emphasizes determining and achieving personal and occupational interests through meaningful activities. It encourages goal setting for personal enrichment. This dimension is linked to the creation of a positive attitude about personal and professional abilities and development. It includes these actions:

- ▶ Engage fully in life
- ▶ Participate in hobbies or an occupation
- ▶ Recognize abilities
- ▶ Identify a personal mission and goals
- ▶ Learn new skills
- ▶ Maintain interests and develop new interests

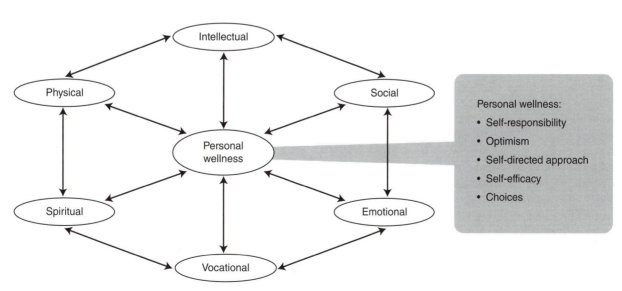

▶ **Figure 1.5** Whole-person wellness wheel.

Whole-person Wellness Model © 1994, Jan Montague.

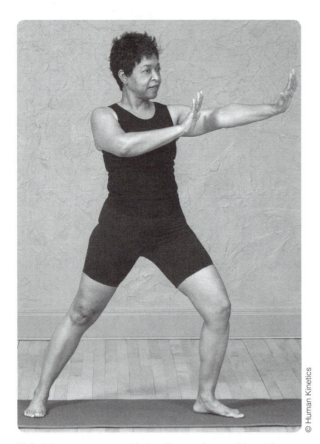

© Human Kinetics

Tai chi engages multiple dimensions of health.

ADULT WELLNESS: THE BIG PICTURE

Changing demographics, the focus on physical activity as preventive medicine, altered expectations of advanced age, changing needs of adults, and awareness of the importance of whole-person health are all factors feeding the tremendous growth in the senior wellness market. A great deal can be accomplished by engaging the fitness industry, senior housing industry, community health agencies, and aging organizations in the quest for wellness. But to be successful, wellness specialists must take heed of behavior change research. Prochaska and Marcus' (1994) original behavior change model identifies five stages of change: precontemplation (not thinking about changing), contemplation (thinking but not ready), preparation (gathering information, intending to change), action (attending a program, changing behavior), and maintenance (maintaining the change). Behavior research further demonstrates that only about 20% of people are ready to take action (e.g., attend a wellness offering) at any one time (Dishman, 1994; Benjamin et al., 2005).

As an industry we must move away from the traditional "build it and they will come" approach that treats participants as customers of wellness offerings. This approach appeals primarily to only the 20% of people in the action stage of change. Instead we must provide information and opportunities to people at all levels of change and engage participants as partners in wellness rather than as customers. Chapter 3 (p. 33) offers more information on stages of change, and both chapters 3 and 4 offer strategies to help integrate these concepts into programming.

Fitness Facilities: Still a Largely Untapped Market

The fitness industry has seen tremendous growth in older adult membership. However, few traditional fitness clubs have made a commitment to this market. Reluctant to turn their attention away from the 18- to 28-year-old clientele, many companies offer a few classes targeting "seniors" but generally retain the standard youth-oriented environment. Physical function and special health conditions affect exercise capacity and safety much more than age, yet many facilities retain the limiting, age-based approach to classes.

Traditional fitness facilities are most likely to attract physically independent adults interested in improving health, physically fit adults working to retain high levels of fitness, and physically elite adults training for competition. Most clubs are ill equipped to provide programming for physically frail and physically dependent adults, although some clubs are incorporating physical therapy programs into their business models. This can be an effective model when therapists work closely with trainers to transition from therapeutic exercise to lifestyle activity.

One significant change in the fitness industry is that new companies are specifically focused on meeting the needs of deconditioned clients, regardless of age. These companies focus on functional ability and actively address more than the physical needs of clients. These centers tend to be smaller and more personalized and acknowledge the importance of developing body confidence and self-efficacy in relation to physical activity behavior.

Senior Housing: Evolution to Wellness

Ten years ago wellness programs in senior housing were defined primarily by regular chair-exercise classes and health management efforts like medical screenings and blood pressure checks. Activity programs were largely driven by the need to fill time slots with activities, but programmers had a difficult time engaging the majority of residents. Progressive senior-living companies are now designing wellness programs using the six-dimensional model of health, including physical, social, emotional, spiritual, intellectual, and vocational well-being.

One significant challenge in senior housing is overcoming the medical model approach, which emphasizes physical well-being as the most important aspect of health. Another challenge is integrating wellness strategies throughout all aspects of the community so all staff, regardless of their primary responsibility, actively support a wellness environment. There are tremendous opportunities in senior-living environments for people who can engage residents as partners in health rather than as customers of wellness offerings. Refer to chapter 7 for specific strategies.

Community Programs and Aging Organizations

Community programs are often challenged to provide programs for the broadest range of functional abilities. The five levels of functional ability and their corresponding immediate needs will help professionals provide safe and effective programs in this market (see chapter 4, p. 53). Community recreation centers and senior centers often focus primarily on physical fitness. However, this market is also incorporating programs like tai chi and yoga that address needs of participants in body, mind, and spirit.

Aging organizations such as the Administration on Aging, National Council on Aging, and American Society on Aging have turned their attention toward helping mature adults stay well. Disease management and prevention programs are being widely disseminated, and as innovative wellness programs gain more national attention, the aging organizations will begin driving the transition to whole-person wellness.

Wellness Leaders: Challenges and Opportunities

Increasing numbers of adults recognize the importance of retaining vitality throughout the life span, and a broad cross-section of organizations are working to ensure that adults have access to programs supporting healthy, active lifestyles. This market growth provides challenges and opportunities for health promotion and wellness specialists.

The first challenge is what to call this new industry. *Senior health promotion* and *senior wellness* imply an age-based approach. Age is only one factor in the equation and has less to do with what a person is capable of than factors such as current level of functional ability, lifestyle habits, attitudes, expectations, and personal beliefs. *Health promotion* fails to capture the breadth of the industry or acknowledge the six dimensions of wellness. So far in this book I have used the term *adult health promotion and wellness*, which is rather cumbersome. Thus, for the remainder of this book I refer to the efforts to improve older adult health in both community and senior-living environments simply as the *adult wellness industry*.

Another challenge is assessing participants' current levels of functional ability and determining whether participants need specialized programming. Chapter 2 provides information on medical conditions that pose safety concerns and offers guidelines to address issues such as diminished vision or hearing, significant muscle weakness, and compromised balance. It is also important to help participants identify their wellness goals and what motivates them to attend class. Their motivation could be to maintain function and a positive quality of life, foster social connections, prepare for vigorous competition, improve appearance, or accomplish something entirely unique. Chapter 4 (p. 51) provides information about simple field-based assessments to determine functional status.

Professionals wishing to branch out into mature-market niches associated with healthy lifestyles will find many new opportunities. The travel and leisure industry has experienced significant growth as a result of aging demographics, and the fastest-growing segments are adventure travel and wellness vacation packages catering to active adults. Adult wellness specialists who can program for multiple levels of functional ability in unique environments will be an important part of this growth industry.

There are opportunities for personal fitness trainers who specialize in helping adults who are competing in sports events or training regularly in order to excel in physically active interests. Personal trainers who specialize in adult wellness can help people prepare for the physical demands of adventure travel and provide well-designed programs for maximum health and vitality. In addition, instructors are needed who can educate other professionals on exercise techniques for clients with special needs. The opportunities for professionals to make a difference in the adult wellness industry are numerous. These professionals will likely find it personally rewarding to offer programs that significantly improve people's quality of life.

WELLNESS WRAP-UP

Population demographics and changing attitudes about aging drive the senior wellness industry. Senior fitness programs must evolve to meet the needs of people at various levels of functional ability, and programming choices must be driven by functional status rather than age. Programs must incorporate all aspects of well-being, including physical, social, emotional, intellectual, spiritual, and vocational dimensions. Senior wellness professionals must work with the fitness industry, senior housing industry, community-based programs, health agencies, and aging services organizations to ensure they have current information to promote well-being among older adults.

The first edition of this book in 1995 focused on exercise. This second edition incorporates what I have learned from years of experience. To maximize well-being for adults, professionals must open many doors into this thing we call wellness. Many adults will never enter wellness programming through the "physical activity" door. But they just might enter through a program focused on emotional or intellectual well-being. Every program, regardless of its main focus, can integrate multiple dimensions.

CHAPTER 2

Exercise Science and Changes in Functional Ability

To work safely and effectively with adult exercisers, you must understand the principles of exercise science. This understanding should include the principles of exercise physiology and how they apply to exercise training, the functional systems of the body and how they interact, and the musculoskeletal structure and how it interacts with the body's other systems to create movement. It is an advantage to have a background in health or physical education that provides some depth of knowledge in the area of exercise science. Although there is no substitute for a thorough understanding, some good resources are available that can help you develop a strong foundation. *Exercise for Older Adults* (Bryant and Green, 2005) and *Physical Activity Instruction of Older Adults* (Jones and Rose, 2005) provide clear, concise explanations of important elements of physiology and of anatomy and kinesiology.

This chapter provides a brief overview of exercise science principles to give you a starting point for further investigation. Do not be intimidated about seeking further knowledge in these important areas. Aggressively expanding your knowledge base will help you ensure that the exercises you offer participants are safe and effective.

In addition to providing information on exercise science, this chapter explains the distinction between *primary aging*, which is aging that occurs with the passage of time, and *secondary aging*, which encompasses the changes associated with lifestyle habits, injury or disease, and the environment. In the past, diminished capacity in the cardiopulmonary, nervous, and musculoskeletal systems observed in older adult populations was blamed on primary aging. But current research shows that although some changes are associated with primary aging, the vast majority of decline is closely linked to a lack of physical activity and other negative lifestyle factors (secondary aging) (Bylina et al., 2006; Chodzko-Zajko, 2005).

The chapter describes common health conditions that affect exercise safety, including hypertension, cardiovascular and pulmonary dysfunction, arthritis, osteoporosis, and diabetes. The chapter then briefly outlines exercise modifications for each condition and suggests resources for further study. Finally, the chapter describes how to address the needs of clients who have prior injuries or are severely deconditioned.

EXERCISE PHYSIOLOGY AND AGING SYSTEMS

Exercise physiology is the study of how the body functions during exercise. It provides the basis for understanding how the body functions at rest and how these functions change during exercise. It also provides an understanding of how the body adapts to exercise training. Exercise physiology examines these functions at the cellular level, which helps us understand the different metabolic systems. An important principle for the fitness instructor to understand is the principle of specificity. Very generally, this principle of training states that physiological adaptations (i.e., changes brought about by exercise) are specific to the systems that are overloaded or stressed with exercise. For example, aerobic metabolism requires a constant supply of oxygen, so aerobic exercise must consist of the types of movement that can be performed continuously over a relatively long period of time without creating oxygen deprivation. Anaerobic metabolism, on the other hand, does not require a replenishment of oxygen and is characterized by quick, explosive movements that can only be performed for relatively short periods of time. To use running as an example, the principle of specificity dictates that if you wish to develop cardiorespiratory endurance, you must provide movements that maintain a constant supply of oxygen, such as jogging, thus allowing aerobic metabolism. If you wish to develop the ability to perform fast, explosive actions, you must provide movement that requires anaerobic metabolism, such as sprinting. Exercise programming designed to maintain the level of aerobic fitness necessary to enjoy a positive quality of life uses movement that calls for aerobic rather than anaerobic metabolism.

Another example of specificity is that to improve muscle strength in the upper body, you must exercise those muscles against resistance (e.g., through weightlifting). Low-impact aerobics or other exercises that use the upper body during exercise may improve muscle endurance somewhat, but to achieve significant gains in strength, the muscles of the upper body must be overloaded or stressed with exercise.

Cardiopulmonary System

The cardiovascular system, composed of the heart and the blood vessels, circulates blood throughout the body. The heart is a muscle that becomes stronger through regular aerobic exercise. A stronger heart muscle is a more efficient pump, requiring less frequent contractions to circulate the amount of blood that the body requires to function. Aerobic exercise also benefits the blood vessels by helping them maintain their essential elasticity and increasing the number of capillaries. The capillaries receive the blood from blood vessels and distribute it to the tissues.

The pulmonary system consists of the lungs and the respiratory tract. The lungs receive blood from the heart and fill the blood with oxygen (from inhaled air). Then the carbon dioxide is carried off and expelled through the respiratory tract (exhaled). The work that the cardiovascular system and the pulmonary system do together to provide oxygen to the rest of the body is called the *cardiopulmonary* or *cardiorespiratory* function.

Changes Over Time

The reduced function of the cardiopulmonary system commonly observed in older people has been associated with a number of important factors. One factor is the diminished level of oxygen transfer. This is related to changes in respiratory function associated with a loss of elasticity of the lung tissue, rigidity of the chest wall, and decreased strength in the respiratory muscles. This combination of conditions contributes significantly to a decrease in cardiopulmonary endurance (Spirduso et al., 2005). Other factors are a decrease in both stroke volume (the volume of blood pumped from the heart during one heartbeat) and maximum heart rate (the highest heart rate a person can attain). The decline in maximum heart rate is estimated to be approximately 5 to 10 beats per decade of age from its peak around age 20. However, maximum heart rate is not predicted well by age alone, and habitual aerobic exercise has a significant impact on maintaining cardiopulmonary endurance (Morgenthal and Shephard, 2005). Decreases in stroke volume and maximum heart rate contribute to diminished cardiac output (the amount of blood pumped by the heart per minute). Finally, there are increases in blood pressure (the pressure exerted by the blood on the walls of the arteries) and other vessel-related difficulties (Spirduso et al., 2005). All of these factors contribute significantly to the decline of performance in cardiopulmonary endurance activities. Again, although age is a factor in some changes in cardiorespiratory function, lifestyle factors contribute most dramatically to the outcome.

Benefits of Exercise

Regular aerobic exercise has been documented to have a significant positive effect on the cardiopulmonary system, slowing and even reversing declines in efficiency that historically were associated with the aging of this system (Boileau et al., 1999; Spirduso et al., 2005). Aerobic exercise is credited with increasing respiratory function, maintaining stroke volume, and reducing resting blood pressure in both young and old participants. Exercise reduces the level of blood lipids and increases glucose tolerance and insulin sensitivity, thus reducing the risk of atherosclerosis and adult-onset diabetes (Hornsby and Albright, 2003). Studies indicate that there is a greater decline with age in the efficiency of oxygen transfer in sedentary people than in those who are physically active. It is clearly documented that exercise has a significant impact on maintenance of aerobic power and endurance. It is encouraging to note that the cardiopulmonary system responds to training regardless of previous physical activity patterns (Spirduso et al., 2005).

Nervous System

The nervous system acts as a computer, controlling all bodily functions. The nervous system consists of the central nervous system (the brain and spinal cord) and the peripheral nervous system (pairs of nerve branches originating from the central nervous system). As the nerves branch out, they continue to subdivide until they integrate with the muscle. The last nerve fiber has branches that attach to the skeletal muscle fibers and stimulate the muscle to contract (Masoro, 1999).

Changes Over Time

The nervous system sends and receives all messages processed by the body and is responsible for the actions resulting from these messages. Aging has a significant impact on the nervous system. It becomes less efficient, and the processes of receiving, processing, and transmitting messages become slower. This results in a slower reaction to these messages. It also seems that a less efficient nervous system has an increased reliance on reactive control (using feedback to initiate corrective movement) rather than predictive control (initiating movement in anticipation of a change). Many older or sedentary people gradually lose the option of predictive control, forcing them to rely only on reactive control. These changes as well as changes in the ability to integrate sensory information contribute to a decline in the ability to efficiently perform tasks requiring speed (Spirduso et al., 2005; Stelmach and Goggin, 1989).

The reduced speed of response holds considerable practical importance, because rapid responses are needed to adequately perform many tasks, such as operating motor vehicles, participating in recreational activities, and preventing falls (Morgenthal and Shephard, 2005). Any decline in sensory perception, such as vision and hearing, will further diminish reaction time. Declines in reaction time, movement time, predictive control, and sensory perception are all responsible for the decline of coordination, balance, and agility often associated with aging. However, physical activity has a dramatic impact on retaining function of the nervous system.

Benefits of Exercise

Regular exercise minimizes the slowing of reaction and movement times. Studies by Stelmach and Goggin (1989a), Smith and Gilligan (1989), and Boileau and colleagues (1999) have demonstrated that physically trained seniors have much faster reaction times than untrained seniors and that faster reaction times can be gained through practice. Aerobic exercise training in previously sedentary older adults can improve many neuropsychological functions, such as response time, visual organization, memory, and mental flexibility (Hall et al., 2001; Spirduso et al., 2005). Research clearly cites physical activity as a powerful intervention for retaining functional capacity of the central nervous system (Christensen et al., 2003; Hall et al, 2001).

Musculoskeletal System

The skeletal system consists of the bones, their articulations (joints), and the tendons and ligaments that hold each articulation together. All movements of the skeletal system take place at the articulations. The muscular system consists of the muscles and their tendinous attachments and provides the forces that cause the bones to move. Each muscle is attached to at least two bones and crosses one or more joints. The interaction of the skeletal system and the muscular system creates a musculoskeletal lever system, which allows movement to occur (Kreighbaum, 1987).

If you visualize the skeleton as a puppet with the muscles as the strings, it will help you understand how the lever system creates movement. Consider how a puppet string can only pull the puppet parts through a movement (such as pulling an arm up until it is parallel with the floor) or control the effects of gravity on a part (such as slowly lowering the raised arm to the side instead of allowing it to drop forcefully). Clearly, a string cannot push a puppet part through movement; likewise, the muscles cannot push the skeleton through movement. Muscles can do only one of two things: (1) shorten or contract to pull the bone through movement (concentric contraction) or (2) attempt to shorten in response to some other resistive force, such as gravity. In the latter case, their attempt to shorten is thwarted by the larger force, and thus the muscle stretches out or lengthens against the resistance (this is termed *eccentric contraction*).

A working knowledge of this system is essential to understanding which muscles are responsible for the movements of each body part. This knowledge will allow you to create an exercise program using "movement that matters" for participants. For example, the quadriceps muscle helps people get up from and sit down on chairs, to walk, and to climb stairs. To exercise the quadriceps you must know that it is responsible for extension (increasing the angle) of the knee joint. Therefore, exercises that extend (straighten) the knee joint will use the quadriceps. Creating additional resistance against extension, such as adding a weight to the ankle, will make the quadriceps work harder to extend the knee, thus contributing to improved strength. Similarly, the hamstring muscle is responsible for flexion (decreasing the angle) of the knee joint. Therefore, exercises that flex (bend) the knee joint will use the hamstring.

Changes Over Time

Reduced efficiency of the musculoskeletal system is related to a number of factors. Diminished muscular strength, power, and endurance are partially attributed to a decrease in the number, size, and type of muscle fibers commonly present in the older adult (Brunner et al., 2007). There is additional evidence that over time and with lack of training, the muscle fibers respond more slowly to nerve stimulation and with a less efficient muscle reflex (Brunner et al., 2007). For sedentary people, changes in the musculoskeletal system result in an average strength loss of about 1% to 1.5% per year from age 50 to 70 and about 3% per year after age 70 (Spirduso et al., 2005). Severe loss of muscle mass and strength even in a relatively small muscle group can result in loss of functional independence. For example, those with low ankle strength have a higher risk of falling (figure 2.1).

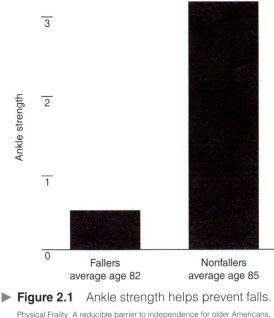

Ankle strength

Fallers
average age 82

Nonfallers
average age 85

▶ **Figure 2.1** Ankle strength helps prevent falls.

Physical Frailty: A reducible barrier to independence for older Americans, 1990. National Institute on Aging.

Recent research has shown that the loss of muscle power (the ability to produce force quickly) happens even more quickly than the loss of strength and is also more closely linked with functional performance than strength alone. Therefore, loss of power has a profound impact on functional independence (Hazell et al., 2007). See chapter 5 for more information about the difference between strength and power.

Another characteristic of an inefficient musculoskeletal system is the general loss of muscle mass, which contributes to the overall decline in lean body mass (i.e., the mass of the body—muscles, bones, nerves, skin, and organs—excluding the fatty tissue). The loss of lean body mass contributes to the decline in basal metabolic rate (the minimum energy required to maintain life processes in a resting state), which in turn contributes to the increase in stored body fat (Spirduso et al., 2005).

Muscle flexibility can demonstrate a marked decline. This decline is influenced by decreases in muscle fiber flexibility and the elasticity of connective tissue (Holland et al., 2002). In addition, there is a decline in joint flexibility and stability relating to changes in the joint components of cartilage, ligaments, and tendons (MacRae, 1986; Spirduso et al., 2005). Without active intervention, the overall loss of flexibility attributed to aging of the muscles

and joints is estimated at 25% to 30% by age 70 (Elkowitz and Elkowitz, 1986). Spirduso and colleagues (2005) cited research indicating a loss of flexibility (measured by the sit-and-reach test) of 15% per decade.

The final factor associated with an aging musculoskeletal system is the decline of the structural integrity of this system, most significantly affected by a decline in bone mass and bone mineral content. Bone loss in both males and females is reported to begin around age 30 with a loss of about 1% per year to age 50. In females, bone loss increases to about 2% to 3% per year after menopause (Spirduso et al., 2005). This higher rate of bone loss in women contributes to the higher rate of osteoporosis and bone fractures among older women. Adult bone health is primarily determined by peak bone mass as a young adult and rate of bone loss with advancing age, which is influenced by sex, ethnicity, hormones, diet, exercise, and body weight.

Benefits of Exercise

Extensive research documents exercise-induced improvements in the musculoskeletal system (Hazell et al., 2003). These improvements include increases in muscular strength, muscular endurance, lean body mass, joint flexibility, and bone mineral content.

Muscular strength, power, and endurance can be increased through training. It is interesting to note that the hypertrophy (increase in muscle size) normally observed in the trained muscle mass of a young person is not as exaggerated in an older person. Therefore, improved strength in the older person may be largely due to the increased ability to recruit motor units (a motor neuron and all of the muscle fibers it activates) observed in the trained muscle of an older adult (Spirduso et al., 2005). Power training has recently gained a significant amount of attention from researchers. As noted in chapter 1, strength is defined as the amount of force a muscle can produce, power is the amount of force the muscle can produce rapidly (strength × speed). Power is critical to functional independence because the speed component affects one's ability to perform daily activities such as rising from a chair, climbing stairs, walking, or recovering from a near fall. Power training can improve strength as much as can strength training alone but has the added benefit of improving muscle power (Fielding et al., 2002; Hazell et al., 2007; Miszko et al., 2003). See chapter 5 for details on programming to improve strength and power.

Exercise helps prevent and restore the loss of muscle mass. It also can reduce fat accumulation, which is closely linked with loss of lean body mass and the resultant decline in basal metabolic rate (Spirduso et al., 2005). Stamford (1988) indicated that a person's level of body fat is much more closely connected to habitual levels of physical activity than to age. Physical activity, even when initiated late in life, can bring about positive changes in body composition.

Research clearly documents how regular physical activity can maintain and improve muscle flexibility (Holland et al., 2002). Studies have recorded similar improvements in flexibility between young and older participants who participate in the same training programs (Smith and Gilligan, 1989a). MacRae (1986) reported improvements in flexibility in participants who were involved in a nonstrenuous progressive program as well as in those involved in a more strenuous jogging and cycling program.

Exercise plays a critical role in maintaining a strong, efficient musculoskeletal system, which promotes lifelong functional independence and quality of life. Inactivity and the resultant lack of mechanical force applied to bones are key factors in bone changes and bone loss (Spirduso et al., 2005). When bone loss declines to such a level that fractures occur with minimal trauma, the integrity of the musculoskeletal system is severely diminished. This weakened state of bone is called *osteoporosis* and is responsible for a high percentage of fractures in older women (Bloomfield and Smith, 2003). Weight-bearing exercise, especially resistance training, has been proven to help prevent bone loss and increase bone mineral content, contributing to the prevention of osteoporosis (Hawkins et al., 2002; Spirduso et al., 2005).

PHYSICAL CONDITIONS REQUIRING SPECIAL CONSIDERATION

Several health conditions that affect exercise potential and safety occur at a high rate in the older adult population and require exercise modifications to ensure safe participation. Next I discuss some of the most frequently encountered conditions and those that can most significantly compromise the safety of your exercise program. An excellent resource for many chronic conditions is *ACSM's Exercise Management for Persons With Chronic Diseases and Disabilities* (Durstine and Moore, 2003). In addition, the Administration on Aging (www.aoa.gov) and the U.S. Centers for Disease Control and Prevention (www.cdc.gov) have a variety of resources on managing chronic conditions. Readers may also visit www.kayvannorman.com for information on 30-minute seminars designed to help older adults live well with chronic conditions.

Hypertension

Hypertension, or high blood pressure, is prevalent in most Western industrialized countries, especially in adults aged 65 and over (Gordon, 2003; MacRae, 2005). Hypertension ranges from stage 1 (140/90) to stage 3 (180/110). It afflicts close to two thirds of Americans over the age of 65 and is a primary risk factor in heart disease, coronary artery disease, and stroke (Rimmer, 2005a). In 95% of people being treated for hypertension there is no identifiable cause, but those with hypertension are reported to be at significantly higher risk for a stroke and congestive heart failure than those without hypertension (Gordon, 2003). A blood pressure reading of 160 or more over 95 may indicate difficulty in the ejection phase of the cardiac cycle. This may be related to decreased arterial elasticity, which results in increased resistance during the systolic (ejection) phase (Hagberg, 1988).

Benefits of Exercise

A gradual increase in blood pressure associated with aging appears to be largely connected to an increasingly inactive lifestyle. Studies demonstrate that endurance exercise produces a significant decrease in both diastolic and systolic blood pressure (Rimmer, 2005b). Aerobic exercise has been consistently shown to offer substantial benefits for older people with hypertension (Hagberg et al., 2000). Medicine-induced declines in blood pressure to the same levels produced by regular endurance exercise are associated with a 20% to 60% decline in mortality and morbidity. The additional benefit of exercise is its positive effect on the reduction of other risk factors associated with cardiovascular disease (Hagberg, 1988).

Exercise Modifications

The cardiac response to exercise in a hypertensive population varies according to the level of hypertension, medication, and individual differences. Low- to moderate-intensity exercise (40-70% of maximum heart rate) for 30 to 60 minutes 3 to 7 days per week appears to be very beneficial. Studies indicate that low-intensity aerobic exercise appears to lower blood pressure as much as, and in some cases more than, higher-intensity exercise (Goldberg and Hagberg, 1990; Gordon, 2003). Low- to moderate-intensity exercise reduces blood pressure while putting the hypertensive exerciser at a much lower risk for cardiac difficulties.

Isometric contraction exercises (in which the muscle is strongly contracted without movement of the joint) are shown to increase systolic and diastolic blood pressure and therefore are not the best choice for hypertensive people. Exercises such as resistance training, which provides significant benefits in other areas, can be approached with caution by using low resistance with high (minimum of 20) repetitions (Gordon, 2003). Proper breathing should be emphasized to prevent the increase in blood pressure that occurs if a person holds her breath while exercising against resistance.

Determine whether clients have hypertension and, if so, whether it is being controlled by medication when necessary. Monitor blood pressure more frequently to document the impact of exercise on blood pressure readings. Use the rating of perceived exertion (RPE) to monitor exercise intensity due to the impact of heart rate medications on heart rate responses to exercise. See chapter 4 for more information on the rating of perceived exertion.

Hypertension Medication

Medications used to treat hypertension include β-blockers, calcium channel blockers, and diuretics. Some blockers affect cardiac response by limiting the heart rate; some are vasodilators, which decrease peripheral resistance in the blood vessels; and some affect both. Because β-blockers artificially regulate the heart rate, medicated exercisers must learn to accurately assess their rating of perceived exertion during exercise. Diuretics increase urine output, which may cause participants on those medications to restrict fluid intake before exercise class. Encourage all clients to drink plenty of fluids before and after exercise to prevent dehydration.

Several studies show that β-blockers can decrease the capacity for prolonged endurance exercise (Goldberg and Hagberg, 1990; Wilmore, 1988). This may have implications in the duration of aerobic exercise appropriate for a person with hypertension. Other studies indicate that β-blockers may also have a negative effect on thermoregulation, making those on such medication more susceptible to temperature extremes (Wilmore, 1988). Avoid having people with hypertension exercise in extreme heat, which could increase stress on the cardiovascular system.

Heart rate medications invalidate exercise heart rate calculations. Clients on heart rate medications should not try to reach a target heart rate but instead must use the RPE to gauge exercise intensity. For this reason, even nonmedicated clients should use RPE in conjunction with heart rate calculations to improve safety for people who may have an undiagnosed condition. See chapter 4 for specific information on RPE and other methods of monitoring exercise intensity.

The time exercise is performed in relation to when the medication is taken is a significant factor. The body's response to exercise will vary according to how close exercise is performed to the peak response time (i.e., when the drug is having its maximum effect) (Bloomfield and Smith, 2003). Consider this factor when performing formal exercise testing. For example, if exercise is normally performed 1 hour after the client takes the medication, then an exercise test should also be performed 1 hour after taking medication. Relay to your participants the significance of the timing of medication use in relation to the performance of exercise. Consistent timing between medication and aerobic exercise will increase the accuracy of the rating of perceived exertion.

Cardiovascular and Pulmonary Disease

Cardiovascular disease is the leading cause of disability and death in the United States (CDC, 2007). Many older adults will exhibit some form of cardiovascular disease resulting from a variety of risk factors involving heredity and lifestyle. *Cardiovascular disease* is a broad term that can refer to a wide range of disorders of the cardiovascular system. Pulmonary disease relates to disorders affecting the respiratory system, including emphysema, bronchitis, and asthma. All cardiovascular and pulmonary diseases have some implication for exercise programs, especially those that include aerobic conditioning.

Benefits of Exercise

Exercise helps prevent heart disease and is also an important aspect of recovery from the functional losses resulting from heart disease (MacRae, 2005). Heart attack survivors will begin their recovery in cardiac rehabilitation programs connected to hospital settings that facilitate the careful monitoring of exercise intensity and response necessary in this population. An older adult with pulmonary dysfunction can also benefit from exercise. Regular exercise may not provide a significant increase in pulmonary function, but it will help decrease respiratory symptoms and can also decrease anxiety and depression related to illness. Exercise can also improve one's ability to perform activities of daily living (ACSM, 1991b).

Exercise Modifications

An exercise program focusing on low- to moderate-intensity exercise may be appropriate for patients in the final stages of recovery from cardiac disease. However, such people should participate in aerobic exercise only under the careful guidance of their physicians, who must determine the appropriate level of exercise intensity and monitor participants' progress. Those with pulmonary dysfunction must also modify the duration and frequency of exercise to allow for respiratory restrictions. For example, if 20 to 30 minutes of continuous exercise is unattainable, two 10- to 15-minute exercise sessions or even four 5-minute sessions may be appropriate (Durstine and Moore, 2003). Even when the duration must be modified considerably, exercise is still beneficial and should be pursued by those with cardiovascular and pulmonary disorders.

Arthritis

According to the Arthritis Foundation, the word *arthritis* means joint inflammation and refers to a host of rheumatic diseases. Inflammation is characterized by swelling, pain, stiffness, and redness and can occur to varying degrees in the joints, muscles, and connective tissues of the body. Arthritis significantly limits the range of motion in the joints. It is considered a chronic condition (i.e., one having no cure) but can be managed through proper treatment programs.

Osteoarthritis is a progressive, irreversible form of arthritis characterized by degeneration of the articular surfaces of the joint. It usually involves continuous discomfort and affects weight-bearing joints, such as knees, hips, and spine. It begins most often after age 40. Rheumatoid arthritis is a common inflammatory arthritis that can cause severe damage and usually affects many joints. It involves periods of acute pain during flare-ups and periods of little or no pain during remission. It can occur at any age and more commonly affects women (Minor and Kay, 2003).

Water Exercise Is My Lifeline

Bev has rheumatoid arthritis. This excerpt from a letter she wrote expresses what arthritis water exercise has done for her: "After spending over 2 years trying every medicine known without positive results, I wound up in a wheelchair. Then I discovered water exercise when I came to live with my daughter, who happened to be teaching for the Bozeman Young at Heart program. It truly was a turning point in my life. In 6 weeks I was out of the wheelchair. When I thought I was doing pretty well I moved back to my own town, but unfortunately there was no water exercise program there. Within 2 months I was back in the wheelchair. It was at that point that I knew that water exercise was always going to be a part of my life. I sold my home and moved to Bozeman to become a permanent fixture in the arthritis water exercise program, improving my physical function to a point where I can work 4 days a week."

Bev had a setback when a car accident caused a severe case of whiplash and other back injuries that prevented her from attending classes for almost a year. When she called to tell me that she was finally going to be able to start classes again, she talked about how great it was going to feel to get back in the water and regain her strength and mobility, lose the weight she had gained through the inability to exercise, and bring her arthritis back into check. "These classes are my lifeline," she said.

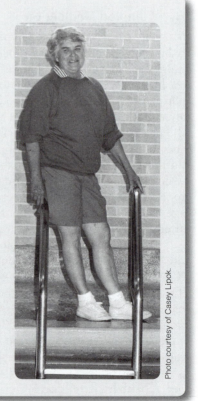

Photo courtesy of Casey Lipok.

Benefits of Exercise

Arthritis is a major crippler in the United States, afflicting almost 43 million U.S. adults (CDC, 2007). Osteoarthritis is considered a degenerative joint disease, and rheumatoid arthritis is considered an inflammatory disease of the immune system reacting against joint tissue. Both forms of arthritis affect exercise safety. Fortunately, appropriate exercise can have a significant impact on controlling the symptoms of arthritis. Regular exercise can help maintain a level of function in the joints that will allow those with arthritis to remain independent.

Exercise Modifications

Include both range of motion and strength exercises in classes designed for those with arthritis. Strengthening exercises can include isotonic resistive exercise (in which the joint is exercising against light weight or some other resistance) or isometric exercise (in which the muscle contracts but does not move the joint). These types of exercise can safely and effectively improve strength, whereas ballistic (jerky or excessive) exercise can aggravate inflammation and harm the joints.

According to the Arthritis Foundation, if a person has exercise-induced pain in the joints that lasts 2 hours or more after exercise, he or she has done too much. Exercisers must learn to recognize their own levels of ability and stop before signs of fatigue appear. Pain in the joint is a warning that the exerciser may be causing further damage to the joints. It is especially critical to adjust exercise during the occasion of arthritic flare-ups. Some flare-ups may require bed rest, passive exercise (someone else gently moving the joint through a range of motion), and direct physician supervision.

Non-weight-bearing exercises, such as water exercise, swimming, chair exercise, and cycling, are well tolerated by those with arthritis. In addition, yoga and Pilates-based programs have proven to be beneficial for this population (Larkin, 2007). While developing exercise sequences, alternate more difficult activities with easier ones to minimize fatigue. Encourage class participants to plan ahead for exercise class by not overexerting themselves before class. Continually emphasize the importance of each person working at his or her own level of ability. Avoid the use of positions that can lead to joint deformity, such as tight grips on objects or the side of the pool during water exercise. Finally, weigh the risks to the joint with the benefits provided by the movement. For example, although a weight added to the ankle during knee extensions will increase muscle strength, if it causes pain to an already compromised knee joint it should not be used.

One good resource dealing specifically with arthritis and exercise is *The Arthritis Exercise Book*, available from the Cornerstone Library, Simon & Schuster Building, 1230 Avenue of the Americas, New York, NY 10020. For more resources, visit the Arthritis Foundation at www.arthritis.org.

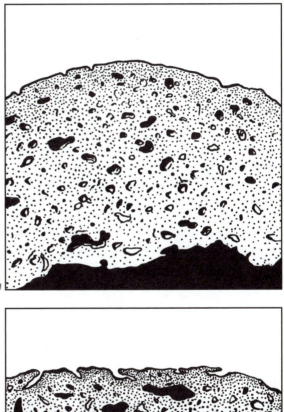

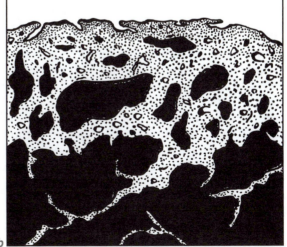

▶ **Figure 2.2** *(a)* Normal and *(b)* osteoporotic bone. Increased dark areas indicate less bone.

Osteoporosis

Osteoporosis is a major public health threat for an estimated 44 million Americans, or 55% of people older than 55, accounting for close to 2 million fractures a year in the United States. In 2005, the fractures occurring with the highest incidence were vertebral at 547,000, followed by wrist fractures at 397,000 and hip fractures at 297,000. Osteoporosis is the loss of bone mineral density to such a degree that fractures can occur after even minimal trauma. Among adults older than 50, an average of 24% of people who sustain a hip fracture die within 1 year (CDC, 2007). A comparison of a healthy bone and an osteoporotic bone is illustrated in figure 2.2 (p. 23).

Factors contributing to osteoporosis are the gradual decline of bone mass associated with the aging skeletal system, the elevated rate of bone loss due to the onset of menopause in women, heredity, and lifestyle factors (smoking, alcohol consumption, poor nutrition, and lack of physical activity) (CDC, 2007). Damage to the skeletal structure caused by osteoporosis cannot be reversed, although some medications appear to improve bone density. Therefore, maximizing bone mass in young adults and preventing bone loss and fractures are very important. The most common avenues of prevention are medication therapy for postmenopausal women, calcium supplementation, and increased physical activity (Rimmer, 2005b). Studies done on young, amenorrheic (nonmenstruating) female athletes demonstrate that estrogen plays the largest role in preventing the decline in bone mineral density; calcium and physical activity are important additions to the treatment.

Benefits of Exercise

Studies have shown that lack of physical activity promotes bone loss. Smith and Gilligan (1989b) reported that the removal or decrease of muscular or gravitational forces on bone segments causes bone atrophy. The degree of atrophy is influenced by the bone's normal role in weight bearing; those bones responsible for greater loads show more rapid atrophy when the load is removed. Increases in bone mineral density are greater in the bones where the force is applied; for example, tennis players often experience significant bone hypertrophy (enlargement) in the dominant arm (Smith and Gilligan, 1989b).

Postmenopausal women are susceptible to osteoporosis because of the increased bone loss associated with the loss of estrogen. Therefore, they are the most common study group for determining the effect of physical activity on bone loss. Studies show that women who exercise regularly will slow bone loss and even gain bone mineral density (Goldberg and Hagberg, 1990; Spirduso et al., 2005). Other studies show that when formerly sedentary subjects participate in a regular physical activity program, bone loss is decreased or bone mineral density is even increased (Smith and Gilligan, 1989b). It is also clear that when exercise is reduced, the loss of bone mineral density resumes. Exercise increases strength, posture, and balance, which can increase functional status and decrease falls and their resultant fractures (Bloomfield and Smith, 2003).

Exercise Modifications

Research clearly shows that to affect the loss of bone mineral density, exercise must be weight bearing (Rimmer, 2005b). Resistance training has been shown to be especially beneficial to help improve bone mineral density, muscle mass, strength, and balance in postmenopausal women. (Nelson et al., 1994). Exercise for prevention of osteoporosis can also include moderate-intensity weight-bearing activities, such as low-impact aerobics and vigorous walking. Avoid ballistic or jarring movements. Also, some positions such as standing for extended times on one leg may place a vulnerable bone at risk. Such exercises should be limited to a maximum of 8 repetitions at a time. For those people who are in the later stages of osteoporosis, exercising while standing on one leg should be avoided completely.

Consider carefully the benefits versus the risks of any vigorous movements. For someone with osteoporosis who is at a high risk of falling, chair exercise and chair-assisted exercise is more appropriate than free-standing exercise. Also, when programming exercise for osteoporotic people, avoid excessive flexion of the spine (i.e., bending forward at the waist), which can contribute to spinal fractures and will place internal organs (already crowded because of osteoporotic-induced spinal changes) in a position vulnerable to injury. Know the visible signs of osteoporosis, such as spinal kyphosis (hunched spine) and pain in common problem zones such as hips, back, and wrists (Rimmer, 2005b). Plan classes that will be safe for people with beginning stages of osteoporosis (often undiagnosed), and seek physician input when creating programs for people with diagnosed osteoporosis.

Diabetes

Diabetes is a condition associated with the body's inability to properly metabolize glucose. When a person ingests food it is changed to glucose, which is carried through the bloodstream for use by the cells. The pancreas responds by secreting the appropriate level of insulin necessary for changing glucose into energy usable by the cells. A person with diabetes is either unable to produce or unable to effectively use insulin (Hornsby and Albright, 2003; Rimmer, 2005b).

There are two main types of diabetes. In type 1, or insulin-dependent, diabetes, the body is either completely unable to produce insulin (which controls blood glucose levels) or produces such a small amount that insulin injections are necessary. In type 2, or non-insulin-dependent, diabetes, the pancreas secretes insulin but the body does not respond effectively to insulin action, and high levels of glucose remain in the bloodstream. People with diabetes (type 1 or type 2) are at greater risk for cardiovascular disease, nerve damage, kidney failure, infections, and eye problems (Barnes, 2004; Gordon, 1993).

Benefits of Exercise

Physical activity has been proven very effective in decreasing the amount of insulin required by injection and increasing the efficiency of the body's response to insulin (i.e., increased insulin sensitivity). Both aerobic exercise and strength training have been shown to assist in managing blood glucose levels and increasing insulin sensitivity. They also help people maintain appropriate body weight (Gordon, 1993; Rimmer, 2005b). Carefully monitor individual responses to exercise to ensure safe, effective exercise programming for those with diabetes.

Exercise Modifications

Have participants undergo a detailed medical evaluation before beginning an exercise program. Put safety at the top of the priority list by following proper exercise protocol such as warming up and cooling down adequately, avoiding exercise in

WARNING SIGNS OF HYPOGLYCEMIA

1. Mild hypoglycemic reaction

- Trembling or shakiness

- Nervousness

- Rapid heart rate

- Palpitations

- Increased sweating

- Excessive hunger

2. Moderate hypoglycemic reaction

- Headache

- Irritability and other abrupt mood changes

- Impaired concentration and attentiveness

- Mental confusion

- Drowsiness

3. Severe hypoglycemic reaction

- Unresponsiveness

- Unconsciousness and coma

- Convulsions

Reprinted, by permission, from N.F. Gordon, 1993, *Diabetes: Your Complete Exercise Guide.* Cooper Clinic and Research Institute Fitness Series (Champaign, IL: Human Kinetics).

adverse climatic conditions without precautions, drinking plenty of fluids, and knowing the warning signs of an impending cardiac complication.

Instruct participants to pay special attention to proper foot care and shoe selection to avoid complications with foot circulation. Participants and instructors should memorize the symptoms of hypoglycemia (see the sidebar) and have an appropriate snack available in case of a hypoglycemic event. Be sure others know where the snack is located. Have participants monitor blood glucose for 12 hours after exercise when beginning a new form of exercise or when making a major change in the intensity or duration of exercise (Barnes, 2004).

Participants can help prevent hypoglycemia by monitoring their blood glucose levels before, during, and after exercise. They should avoid exercising when blood glucose is higher than 250 milligrams per deciliter (type 1) and ketones are present in their urine or when blood glucose is higher than 300 milligrams per deciliter (type 2). They should ask their doctor to help coordinate the insulin regimen with a daily exercise schedule that includes time of day when exercise is performed in relation to insulin dosage, the type and dosage of insulin used, and the duration and intensity of the exercise (Barnes, 2004). Remind participants that hypoglycemia can occur as much as 15 hours after exercise is stopped. Two excellent references for diabetes and exercise are *ACSM's Action Plan for Diabetes* (Barnes, 2004) and *Diabetes: Your Complete Exercise Guide* (Gordon, 1993).

Injury and Disuse

Some clients will have a joint whose movement is compromised because of a severe injury of a muscle, tendon, or ligament. The injury may have occurred many years ago, and the affected muscles simply never received proper rehabilitation. In most cases, the muscle is no longer damaged but, because of disuse, has lost the ability to function properly.

Others may suffer from dysfunction due to extreme muscle weakness resulting from chronic disuse, which is characteristic of a very sedentary lifestyle. Dysfunction caused by the extreme loss of muscle mass is common among those who have been ill and therefore chair-bound or bedridden for an extended period of time. Still, in most cases

of injury or disuse dysfunction, proper exercise can significantly increase the function of the affected joint or muscle.

In the case of an injury-related dysfunction, a physical therapist is the best resource for determining what types of movements are appropriate for the affected joint and muscle segment. With the right kinds of movement, it may be possible to increase the participant's level of function even when the injury is many years old. Exercises that involve some passive movement aid may be beneficial. For example, resistance bands, described in the chair-exercise portion of chapter 5, can be used to aid the affected muscles in completing range of motion exercises.

In extreme cases of muscle weakness or loss of muscle mass due to chronic disuse, seek the advice of a physical therapist. In such cases, the joints can be very unstable because of inflexibility of the tendons and ligaments that surround the joints and the weakness of the muscle tissues that would normally protect the integrity of the joint. The wrong kinds of exercises can pose an unacceptable risk of injury to this weakened structure. Once a physical therapist prescribes the types of movements that are appropriate, you can help your exercise participants accomplish the movement tasks in a variety of ways.

Medications and Exercise

Be aware of the kinds of medication your participants are taking, the potential side effects, and the possible interactions of combined medications. The effects of medication on exercise are as varied as the numbers of medications and the spectrum of individual reactions to medications, so a detailed discussion is beyond the scope of this book. See the following references for more information: Rimmer (2005a), ACSM (1991a), and Durstine and Moore (2003). Make your participants aware of their responsibility in assessing—with their physician—the impact of their medications on exercise safety. Seek the advice of a physician or pharmacist if you have any question about the safety of exercise and a specific medication. Also, be aware that many medications will affect sensory perception, balance, and coordination, so adhere to the guidelines in chapters 4 and 5 for providing safe movements.

WELLNESS WRAP-UP

To create safe and effective exercise programs for adults, you must understand the principles of exercise science and how to apply concepts of exercise training. You must also understand the difference between primary and secondary aging.

You should seek further knowledge in exercise science so you have the background and knowledge to meet the needs of clients with diminished function or chronic conditions affecting exercise potential and safety.

Although this chapter focuses on the physical dimension of wellness, it is important to remain mindful of the wellness approach. Rather than focus on what a client cannot do, focus on what she can do. Seek modifications that allow participants to accomplish their wellness goals, regardless of physical challenges. See chapter 3 for information on how living with a chronic condition can influence a person's belief in her ability to exercise safely.

Psychosocial Aspects of Programming

To create quality programs for adults you must understand more than just the physical aspects of aging and physical activity. Evidence has long suggested that beliefs, assumptions, and expectations can contribute to illness as well as to healing. Now a significant body of research documents that a person's perception of health can powerfully affect physical and psychological symptoms, health choices and behaviors, and ultimately outcomes (Ray, 2004).

Regular exercise improves both physical and mental health and can significantly affect psychological elements of well-being like self-concept, self-efficacy, body image, and mood (Spirduso et al., 2005; Umstattd & Hallam, 2007). Improvements in these elements can, in turn, promote feelings of competence and contribute to higher levels of physical activity (Berger, 1989; Umstattd and Hallam, 2007). With so much to gain from physical activity, it is surprising that the vast majority of adults older than 65 maintain largely sedentary lifestyles (Armstrong et al., 2001; CDC, 2007).

This chapter examines psychosocial aspects of aging and physical activity participation, including elements that create motives for and barriers to physical activity. It also provides practical strategies to help professionals create programs and program messages that positively engage these elements.

UNDERSTANDING PSYCHOSOCIAL CONCEPTS

Perceptions of yourself and perceptions of how you are viewed by others significantly influence your motivation to make changes (Benjamin et al., 2005; Semerjian & Stephens, 2007; Shephard, 1999). The following factors can affect one's motivation to change:

- Attitudes toward behavior
- Perceived norms for behavior
- A person's belief that certain referents (e.g. doctor, spouse, friend) think she should or shouldn't perform behavior
- Motivation to comply (or not) with perceived wishes
- Belief that change is positive
- Belief that action taken will result in desired change (Shephard, 1999)

Expectations, attitudes, subjective norms, and perceived behavioral control are other psychosocial elements related to physical activity participation and outcomes. I use the general term *personal beliefs* when referring to how these elements combine to determine a person's view of the world and his overall perceived competence and place in the world.

Perceptions of Self

Perception of self is influenced by a long list of internal and external factors. Researchers have identified self-efficacy, self-concept, and self-esteem as significant contributors to self-perception (Spirduso et al., 2005). Each factor plays a role in determining a person's body confidence, social competence, perceptions of abilities, and perceived behavioral control (how much control a person believes he has over performing a behavior). These factors also affect whether a person feels positive about his life and circumstances, and research is being conducted to explore what role the field of positive psychology can have on older adult well-being (Coalman, 2007). Perceptions of self and of life circumstances affect a person's physical activity behavior.

- **Self-efficacy** is defined as a person's perceived confidence in her ability to perform a specific behavior in a given setting (Umstattd & Hallam, 2007). In regard to exercise behavior, self-efficacy refers to one's perceived confidence to overcome barriers to exercise (Bandura, 1997). Numerous studies have identified self-efficacy as both a key element in predicting physical activity behavior and a positive outcome of physical activity participation (Cheung et al., 2006; Lucidi et al., 2006; Umstattd & Hallam, 2007). A person considering participation in an exercise program will evaluate the program components and estimate her ability to be successful in the program. She will enroll in the program only if she believes she will be successful in most or all of the components (Spirduso et al., 2005). Chapter 4 provides specific strategies to ensure success in movement for exercise participants.

- **Self-concept** is defined as the conscious awareness and perception of self. It includes perceptions and evaluations about all aspects of self, including intellectual, social, emotional, spiritual, vocational, and physical function. Self-concept evolves and changes through the various stages of life and includes comparisons with others as well as comparisons with one's own performances at different times (Spirduso et al., 2005). The term *self-concept* is often used interchangeably with *self-esteem*.

■ **Self-esteem,** which is very closely linked with self-concept, consists of the feelings one has about oneself based on evaluations and comparisons of performance. It is the respect and appreciation people have for themselves and includes feelings of competence and self-acceptance (Semerjian & Stephens, 2007; Spirduso et al., 2005). Self-esteem is multidimensional, so a person can have a high level of self-esteem in one area of life and a low level in another area of life.

Perceptions of Aging and Physical Activity

Expectations, attitudes, subjective norms, and perceived behavioral control all affect perceptions of aging and physical activity. They are intertwined with perceptions of self and offer insight into some of the motives for and barriers to physical activity participation.

■ **Expectations** involve what a person believes is the probable outcome of a specific behavior. For example, a person's belief that engaging in physical activity will lead to a certain outcome (like losing weight) is his *outcome expectation*. Expectations can be based on past observations and experiences, information received from the media or other sources, or simply personal beliefs. Expectations about both aging and physical activity play a dominant role in determining health choices, behaviors, and outcomes.

An important aspect of expectations is the *outcome expectancy value*, defined as the interaction between a person's outcome expectation (e.g., losing weight) and how much value he places on that outcome (Umstattd & Hallam, 2007). This value affects a person's ability to commit to a particular course of action and relates to development of self-regulation strategies such as goal setting and self-monitoring of performance.

■ **Attitudes** are favorable or unfavorable evaluations associated with beliefs and behaviors. In the case of physical activity, people may have a positive or negative attitude about exercise based on their experiences or simply based on beliefs and expectations. Negative attitudes about aging are a chief ingredient of *ageism*, which is the tendency to focus disproportionately on any negative aspects of aging (Chodzko-Zajko, 2005). Ageism is defined

as discrimination based on chronological age and includes three elements: prejudicial attitudes toward older people, social or employment discrimination, and policies and procedures that perpetuate aging stereotypes and thereby reduce older people's opportunities for life satisfaction and dignity (Chodzko-Zajko, 2005). Pervasive negative stereotypes and ongoing negative messages about aging can prevent older adults from believing in their ability to effect positive change, especially those with low self-esteem and self-efficacy (Dishman, 1994). Many people with functional limitations or chronic conditions do not perceive themselves as capable of regular physical activity (Benjamin et al., 2005; Rasinaho et al., 2006).

■ **Subjective norms** refer to the perceived social pressure to perform or not to perform a given behavior and can significantly affect a person's physical activity choices (Benjamin et al., 2005). Subjective norms involve one's belief that significant others would either approve or disapprove of the behavior, weighted by the person's motivation to comply or not comply with these referents. Cousins (1997) found that physical activity choices by older adults were often influenced by a person's perception of what is or is not age-appropriate behavior. For example, peers may criticize a person's attempt at regaining fitness as an exercise in vanity or a desire to recapture youth, thereby discouraging participation. In addition, the paternalistic model (doctor as ultimate authority) has dominated health care for many decades, which can discourage people from exerting control over their own health and well-being.

■ **Perceived behavioral control** is the perceived ease or difficulty associated with performing a particular behavior and is influenced by many of the elements discussed. Perceived behavioral control and self-efficacy are both strong predictors of behavioral intention (Lucidi et al., 2006). In the case of physical activity participation, perceived behavioral control includes one's beliefs about the opportunities available to her for physical activity, weighted by the perceived power of factors related to the opportunity that either support or prevent participation (Benjamin et al., 2005). For example, a person may identify an exercise class to attend and then evaluate factors like the time of day and location to determine how easy or difficult it would be to attend. She may also weigh factors such as her spouse's attitude toward her attending the class before making a commitment.

Understanding expectations, attitudes, subjective norms, and perceived behavioral control helps you identify what motivates clients to attend class. Such understanding can also offer insight into what might help a prospective client take action and start attending.

IDENTIFYING PSYCHOSOCIAL BARRIERS

Health promotion specialists have made significant progress identifying and addressing common barriers to physical activity participation, such as transportation, accessibility, cost, environment, and quality programming and staff. However, in retirement communities where none of these identified barriers exist, the majority of residents (often as high as 80%) still remain inactive. Nationwide, 28% of U.S. adults older than 65 report being completely inactive, and 65% fail to meet the U.S. Centers for Disease Control and Prevention physical activity recommendations (Umstattd & Hallam, 2007). I believe that consistently low participation rates in both community-based and senior-living-based venues result from a failure to address psychosocial aspects of physical activity participation (discussed above) and failure to apply behavior change concepts to program design.

Stages of Change

Prochaska's well-documented stages of change theory offers insight into behavior change. He stated that people go through five distinct stages of change when adopting a new behavior: precontemplation, contemplation, preparation, action, and maintenance. Research by Prochaska and Marcus (1994) shows that only about 20% of people with a less-than-ideal behavior are prepared to change (take action) at any one time. In senior-living facilities, the average rate of participation in physical activity classes hovers around 20% to 25%. An even smaller percentage of community-living older adults regularly participate in physical activity classes.

Applying the stages of change theory to physical activity participation demonstrates that standard health promotion strategies have made progress removing barriers for adults in the action stage of change (those who are ready to take action by attending a class) but have done little to move people from precontemplation, contemplation, and preparation into action. Page 33 outlines the five stages of change and also offers programming sug-gestions to match each stage of change. See chapter 7 for more specific programming ideas.

Personal Belief Factors

To move people through the first three stages of change into action (becoming more physically active), we must consider factors that contribute to personal beliefs about aging and physical activity. Generational bias, gender bias, and media images of aging and fitness can form unseen barriers to participation and thus prevent a person from moving from sedentary behavior to a physically active lifestyle. Understanding these factors can help us address and remove them.

Generational Bias

Life-course theory, which posits that the historical times and places people experience over their lifetimes have an influence on their lives (Bradley and Longino, 2001), provides an important perspective on generational bias. This life course shapes a person's personal beliefs, and although vast differences exist among people depending on their personal experiences, important similarities emerge with regard to physical activity.

To effectively deliver the message of wellness to adults at each stage of change, we must understand similarities in the life course of adults older than 60 and how the resulting personal beliefs create the lens through which these people view physical activity programs and program messages.

For example, before today's labor-saving technology, life was much more physically demanding, forging a strong association (for the 60+ generation) between physical activity and the hard physical work necessary both on the job and at home. Time spent in sedentary relaxation was often considered the reward for a hard day's work. I have heard many older adults express a belief in their "earned right" to rest and relax, so, for some, age is the ultimate "pass" from exercise. Unfortunately, few recognize the high price (in functional decline) they will pay for prolonged sedentary behavior.

In addition, adults older than 60 grew up during the era of the industrial revolution, when a good portion of time and energy was devoted to conceiving of ways to remove the burden of physical exertion. Therefore, the perception that physical exertion is undesirable and happily avoidable lingers for many adults. Furthermore, automation and labor-saving devices brought a dramatic and welcome change of lifestyle, but only for those who could afford it.

STAGES OF CHANGE AND MATCHING PROGRAMS

Researcher James Prochaska (Prochaska & Marcus, 1994) identified five hierarchical stages that people typically go through when forming a new habit or changing a behavior. A person's stage of change will determine what messages are relevant to him and what programs will best meet his needs (e.g., increasing physical activity).

Stage	Person's beliefs and actions during stage	Ways the exercise professional can help
Precontemplation	• Does not intend to change or is not ready to change • May not understand the consequences of the behavior or advantages of making the change • May be resistant to change • May view the pros of the negative behavior as greater than the cons	• Give tidbits of information to spark interest. • Provide information that is personally relevant. • Use table tents, flyers, and information cards. • Provide information to people in the general course of their day: Don't require them to go out of their way to receive it.
Contemplation	• Has some knowledge of the consequences or advantages of the change • Believes that the pros and cons of change are about equal • Intends to change or thinks about it but may not know how to get started	• Provide information on physical activity at easily accessible locations. • Attach informational mini-sessions to regularly occurring activities (lunch). • Determine what is personally relevant and address physical activity from that perspective.
Preparation	• Has determined that the pros outweigh the cons • Intends to make a change • Has a plan of action for change within 6 months	• Provide introductory sessions that include a slide show or guest speaker. • Provide resources that allow people to try the exercise on their own. • Organize a workshop, have a sample class, air sessions on a senior living facility's television network, publicize programs in the newspaper. • Make books, brochures, videos, and other activity opportunities easily available.
Action	• Takes action on a regular basis (e.g., attending a class, eating nutritiously) • Tends to feel empowered and in control of life • Has the greatest risk for relapse	• Provide regular classes. • Provide ongoing and easy access to self-directed opportunities (such as stations or videos). • Emphasize goal setting and achievement. • Provide encouragement and reinforcement with ongoing positive messages. • Offer pep talks to prevent relapse.
Maintenance	• Sustains the change for at least 6 months (e.g., walks daily, attends class regularly) • Has abandoned old behavior and wants to prevent relapse • Has made the behavior change part of her lifestyle	• Continue goal setting. • Provide continual access to a variety of opportunities. • Give reinforcement and rewards. • Track progress and improvements. • Introduce new programs and opportunities.

Data from J.O. Prochaska and B.H. Marcus, 1994, The trans-theoretical model: Application to exercise. In *Advances in exercise adherence,* edited by R.K. Dishman (Champaign, IL: Human Kinetics), 161-179.

Automation was new and expensive, forging a strong link between financial success and reduced physical exertion. There was a clear distinction between laborers and "gentlemen" who did little physical work and between housewives and "ladies of the house" who had domestic help. This generation started with the push lawnmower, traded up to the power lawnmower, and moved up further to the riding lawnmower, and when they had really "made it" they could hire someone else to mow the lawn. When filtered through generational bias, the message of physical activity as a positive aspiration is a hard sell to many adults.

Gender Bias

Our cultural climate encourages both males and females to be physically active, including engaging in vigorous sports and other physically challenging activities. However, that has not always been the case. Traditional gender roles and gender bias created both active and passive barriers to physical activity for many adults.

As recently as the 1970s, girls and women were actively discouraged from engaging in recreational exercise. School policies required dresses for girls (unsuited to active play), recognized very few sports as appropriate for girls and women, and failed to fund any female teams, effectively relegating girls to a passive role watching boys play. I personally recall that when girls were first *allowed* to play basketball they were required to play only half-court. The full-court game was considered too vigorous, and vigorous exercise was considered unladylike at best and harmful at worst (to the "weaker" sex). Many women now aged 60+ were, as girls, counseled by physicians and parents to avoid hard physical exertion for fear of damaging reproductive organs.

The perception of exercise as potentially harmful to anyone "delicate" can be pervasive for many adults, even those who believe in the benefits of exercise. This perception can pose a significant barrier to physically frail people or those living with multiple chronic conditions. Current research identifies health problems, fear, and pain as the most commonly perceived barriers to exercise (Cohen-Mansfield et al., 2003; Rasinaho et al., 2007). Benjamin and colleagues (2005) found that physically frail older adults considering exercise were significantly influenced by subjective norms (i.e., the perceived social pressure to perform or not perform a given behavior). For many people, motivation to increase physical activity requires a belief that such a change is desirable, doable, and socially acceptable in light of health status.

Men aged 60+ can also have negative associations related to physical activity. Although boys were encouraged to be more physically active than girls, after a certain age physical activity just for fun was considered a frivolous use of time. A prevailing attitude was that a man with so much time and energy should be doing something productive (Van Norman, 2004). In addition, consider the media images of the 1950s and 1960s showing men coming home from work to be greeted at the door by their wives (with snacks and a newspaper) and encouraged to relax in the easy chair as a reward for a hard day's work.

Many older men also relate fitness to the tough, grueling, and painful exercise they did in military boot camp, concluding that they don't want any part of it, that they can't be successful, that any less vigorous exercise really couldn't do much good anyway, or some combination of these.

Media Images and Expectations

Helping adults change perceptions of exercise is made more difficult by media portrayals of fitness as an extreme. In addition, media images that reinforce negative expectations of aging, or portray a narrow view of successful aging, also make it difficult for many adults to believe in their ability to retain health and vitality throughout the life span.

Perceptions as a Barrier

Nine months pregnant, I arrived to teach a low-impact aerobics class. Participants aged 65 to 75 had been in the Young at Heart exercise program for at least 10 years and were personally committed to physical activity. However, they were appalled, convinced I was going to have the baby right there or injure myself if I didn't stop exercising. This was a significant revelation to me because it translated to "exercise is great for you unless you are in delicate condition, and then it could be harmful."

The media often portrays fitness as exclusive to the "body beautiful" set, portraying an extreme ideal that is completely unrealistic and therefore personally irrelevant to the majority of the population (regardless of exercise habits or diet). Fitness is placed out of reach of the average person, regardless of age, and the consumer culture's preoccupation with perfect bodies and youthful images is especially demeaning to older adults. It creates negative associations with age-related changes and aggressively promotes a belief that these changes are highly undesirable (Bradley & Longino, 2001). This image prevents many people from perceiving themselves as capable of being fit.

The prevailing media image of aging is largely dominated by extremes, effectively reducing older adults to caricatures and leaving them both seriously underrepresented and marginalized by the media (Krueger, 2001). One extreme is characterized by frailty and dependence, spawning endless jokes about aging as well as commercials and sitcoms that portray older adults as nonvigorous, sexless, confused, and a collective drag on social programs and the economy. To complicate matters, much aging research done in the past used subjects who were nursing home residents rather than those who lived independently or even a cross-section of the older adult population. This skewed research sample significantly contributed to the overemphasis of the negative aspects of aging and forged the expectation that most older adults will end up frail and dependent. These portrayals are a cornerstone of *ageism*, which can reduce older people's opportunities for life satisfaction and dignity (Chodzko-Zajko, 2005).

The other extreme showcases "woofies" (well-off older folks), marketed as slender, healthy, financially secure, and at leisure in some fabulous resort community. They are portrayed as the lucky minority who through remarkable genes and large amounts of money and leisure time have escaped the usual consequences of aging. These extremes dominate the media and our perceptions even though it is clear that the majority of older adults exist in the broad range between these extremes. Both negative stereotypes and limited views of successful aging can have a significant impact on the self-esteem, body image, and self-efficacy of older adults. Setting the bar so high or low has significant implications for the perceived range of available and acceptable lifestyle options for adults to relate or aspire to (Bradley and Longino, 2001).

All of the psychosocial elements discussed ultimately determine a person's health beliefs, choices, and behaviors, which in turn affect health outcomes. Wellness specialists who understand and apply the psychosocial elements of exercise behavior to program development can help clients activate the power of the mind–body connection to improve well-being.

APPLYING PSYCHOSOCIAL CONCEPTS

Adults older than 65 are the first generation to experience a dramatically extended life span, but for many it is coupled with multiple chronic conditions. They have enjoyed labor-saving automation but have also discovered the price exacted by inactivity. Few people want to return to a labor-intensive lifestyle, so wellness specialists must reframe intentional physical activity as a positive action rather than something to be avoided. Fortunately, over the past 20 years a great deal of new research has refuted the assertion that aging alone is responsible for dramatic functional declines.

Lifestyle plays a dominant role in one's ability to retain functional independence and quality of life through the full life span (Spirduso et al., 2005), so wellness specialists must educate adults about how much control they have over the physical changes associated with aging (see chapter 2). Instructors must also offer multiple points of entry into wellness programs and consistently work to overcome negative personal beliefs about aging by illuminating common motives for and barriers to physical activity participation.

The six dimensions of wellness (see chapter 1) can help draw people into programming by opening six doors into this thing we call wellness (i.e., physical, social, emotion, intellectual, spiritual, and vocational). Some people may never enter wellness through the physical dimension (e.g., by attending an exercise class). However, they may be interested in programs focused on emotional well-being or intellectual engagement. All programs should strive to engage multiple dimensions to allow a bridge between all six dimensions of well-being. One example of this approach is illustrated by the concept of wellness stations. Wellness stations consist of material posted on walls to allow ongoing, self-directed access to wellness opportunities. Each station demonstrates a physical activity opportunity along with an invitation to engage through another dimension of wellness. One example, Rise to the Occasion (see figure 3.1), addresses the sit-to-stand functional task (physical dimension) and also encourages the participant to actively seek social connections (social dimension). Learn more about how to create wellness stations in chapter 5.

Motivational Triggers and Obtaining Goals

Lees and colleagues (2005) found that nonexercisers usually perceived more barriers to physical activity than exercisers; the top three reasons that people avoided exercise were fear of falling, inertia, and negative effects. Rasinaho and colleagues (2006) found that people with mobility limitations placed a greater emphasis on disease management as a motive for exercise, whereas those without mobility limitations emphasized health promotion. To reframe physical activity as positive, program lead-

ers must understand common motivational triggers and work to increase client self-efficacy for physical activity.

Triggers to attend exercise class are varied and difficult to interpret. It is clear, however, that individual older adults interpret triggers for engaging in exercise very differently. For example, some people will use a perceived threat to health (a common trigger for beginning exercise) to motivate them to exercise, deciding that they need to exercise to regain health. Others will use the same trigger as a barrier to exercise, deciding that they cannot safely exercise because they are ill. This determination will depend on many things, including preconceived notions about the value of exercise, positive or negative expectations, self-efficacy, and level of social support. (O'Brien-Cousins, 2001).

Older adults who choose to participate in physical activity as a response to a trigger generally do so for one or more of the following reasons.

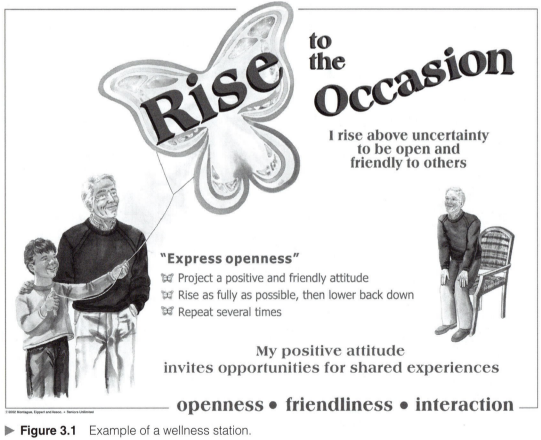

▶ **Figure 3.1** Example of a wellness station.

© Montague, Eippert and Assoc. + Seniors Unlimited.

- They value physical activity as a strategy to obtain a goal.
- They have social support and encouragement to engage in physical activity.
- They believe they can successfully engage in the activity (self-efficacy).
- They have positive expectations that the activity will do them more good than harm (O'Brien-Cousins, 2001).

After participants have taken the first step of joining a program, conduct periodic functional assessments to help them track their progress toward achieving their physical goals. Even if physical accomplishments level off (e.g., when fitness levels plateau), actively addressing the social and emotional elements of class will enhance motivation. Psychosocial rewards such as increases in social connection, increased perception of well-being, and reinforcement of desired self-image can be powerful motivators (Shephard, 1999). Simply having fun can also be a goal and can provide motivation for attending class. Attaining goals and receiving rewards support improved self-efficacy, which is a primary determinant of exercise behavior.

Exercise classes for older adults often become a strong source of social support for participants both inside and outside of class. This social support is an important motivator for attending exercise classes, and increases in social support facilitate increases in self-efficacy (Bandura, 1997).

To help participants develop positive expectations of physical activity, instructors must ensure that the activity addresses needs and takes into account conditions that may put exercisers at risk for injury. This is done by continuously monitoring intensity and suggesting movement modifications for specific conditions. Instructors must also ensure success in movement to support participants' exercise self-efficacy.

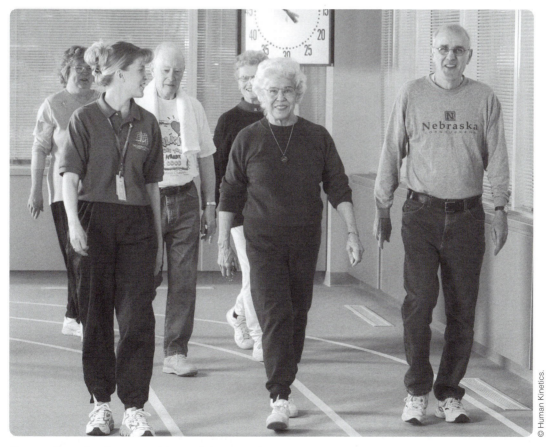

© Human Kinetics.

Connections in class provide social support.

Self-Efficacy and Exercise Behavior

Behavior research identifies self-efficacy as a primary determinant of exercise behavior. Exercise self-efficacy relates to whether a person feels capable of performing exercise to the degree necessary to bring about the desired result (Bandura, 1997). Self-efficacy is such a powerful predictor of behavior that older adults who believe that health is largely biologically ordained are mostly inactive, whereas those who believe that health can be affected by actions taken are significantly more active (Bandura, 1997).

A strong sense of self-efficacy has been found to aid both physical and social recovery from a catastrophic health incidence. In fact, self-efficacy heavily outweighs physical abilities as a determinant for active living after a significant injury or illness (Bandura, 1997). Clearly, a person's belief about her ability to affect her health through actions taken plays a very large role in choices regarding physical activity.

Research by Wise and Trunnell (2001) provides important information about improving self-efficacy. They evaluated the influence of four sources of information on perceptions of self-efficacy:

- Mastery experiences (accomplishing a task)
- Vicarious experiences (watching someone else accomplish a task)
- Verbal persuasion (being told they could accomplish a task)
- Physiological states (changes in physical responses such as heart rate and respiration that signal level of preparation for the task)

Evidence showed that each of these sources is capable of strengthening or weakening perceptions of self-efficacy. The researchers found that successful performance of a task increases self-efficacy more than any other single source. Verbal messages alone had the least effect on self-efficacy. However, specific verbal feedback after successful performance of a task resulted in the greatest increase in self-efficacy. This information supports the validity of ensuring success in movement for all participants and identifying and reviewing goals met as strategies for improving self-efficacy.

A NEW MODEL

The traditional "build it and they will come" model of programming has ensured that people motivated to take action have access to appropriate activities, but it hasn't helped the vast majority of adults become more active. To increase participation, wellness professionals must engage adults as partners in well-being rather than as customers of wellness offerings by using motivation and compliance research to guide program development.

The motivation and compliance research highlights the need for a function-based rather than an age-based approach to programming. It also supports the need for programming approaches that are personally relevant regardless of a person's attitudes toward exercise, perceptions about aging, stage of change, or perceived limitations. Finally, it reinforces the importance of meeting more than just physical needs (i.e., whole-person wellness) and ensuring success, safety, and enjoyment in movement. Wellness specialists must

- recognize how negative stereotypes and media images of aging influence perceived health status, health beliefs, and behaviors;
- understand how personal beliefs about physical activity color perceptions of all physical activity programs and program messages;
- design programs and program messages that are personally relevant to people regardless of their perceptions of aging and physical activity;
- integrate multiple dimensions of health into all programming;
- use psychosocial and behavior change concepts to enhance motivation and compliance; and
- make information and opportunities available not only to participants but also to people who are not yet participants.

One example of how to integrate the psychosocial elements of health and physical activity behavior into physical activity programming, Project MOVE, is described next. The idea behind this approach is to provide research-based and field-tested strategies that engage people at all levels of functional ability and stages of change. It also strives to address multiple dimensions of wellness and offers ways

113% Increase in Strength

Ida Weiss, at 91 years of age, participated in the Fiatarone strength training study through Tufts University in Boston while residing at the Hebrew Rehabilitation Center for the Aged. Subjects aged 72 to 98 participated in a 10-week strength training program that used progressive resistance. Strength increased an average of 113%. Gait velocity and stair-climbing ability also increased significantly (Fiatarone, 1994). In a television interview about strength training, Ida stated, "I didn't think I was going to live anymore, but now I feel different."

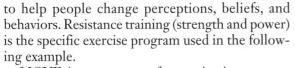

Photo courtesy of Keiser Corporation.

to help people change perceptions, beliefs, and behaviors. Resistance training (strength and power) is the specific exercise program used in the following example.

MOVE is an acronym for motivation, opportunity, verification, and education. Each of these elements plays a role in how successful you will be when introducing a new program. Using the example of strength training, *motivation* refers to helping clients understand why strength and power are personally relevant to them on a daily basis and therefore can affect their quality of life. To motivate people to participate, you must consider generational bias, gender bias, and attitudes and expectations about aging and about strength training when creating programs and program messages. *Opportunity* includes ongoing access to a broad range of resistance training resources and opportunities. You must provide opportunities at multiple levels of functional ability and within multiple dimensions of wellness. In addition, you must create opportunities that will reach people at each stage of change. *Verification* refers to continual reinforcement of the concept that resistance training is desirable, doable, and socially acceptable for people of all functional

abilities. It seeks to normalize the concept and works to affect subjective norms and perceived behavioral control. *Education* involves a systematic approach that delivers both information on resistance training and information designed to change personal beliefs about aging and physical activity. Both verification and education can be supported by newsletters, bulletin boards, seminars, classes, and staff reinforcement of concepts.

Motivation

By now most people are at least aware that resistance training is recommended for improved strength, but people may not believe it applies to them in terms of issues like health status, age, or gender. You must help each client understand how resistance training is personally relevant to her, as in the following examples:

- Use statistics showing the average loss of strength.
- Offer visual representations of the relationship between loss of strength and power and loss of functional independence.

■ Highlight the connections to daily tasks.

■ Offer positive examples of people at various levels of functional status successfully engaging in resistance training.

Research has shown an average strength loss of approximately 1% per year beginning in the early 50s, with much steeper declines, approximately 3% per year, after age 70 (Spirduso et al., 2005). That doesn't sound like much until you do the math. It results in a loss of about 10% by age 60, 20% by age 70, and 50% by age 80. Power is lost at an even greater rate, in some cases as much as four times greater (Hazell et al., 2007). Point out to participants that losing half of one's strength would be roughly the equivalent of going about daily tasks while carrying someone of equal weight on their backs. Figure 3.2 illustrates how a gradual loss of strength affects functional independence.

To make the information more personally relevant, don't just state that resistance training is important; instead relate strength and power research directly to daily functional tasks. For example, say to participants, "You could benefit from becoming stronger if you

■ must use your arms to rise from a chair;

■ struggle to lift sacks of groceries or something off a shelf;

■ hesitate to go places because you are concerned about getting up the steps of the bus, plane, or tourist site;

■ have difficulty doing something that used to be easy; or

■ become easily fatigued when trying to keep up with family or friends."

Most adults cannot imagine losing so much physical function they would be unable to manage the activities of daily living, yet many currently independent but sedentary older adults are only one or two illnesses or injuries away from dependence. To ensure personal relevance, ask potential clients important questions:

■ "One year from now, do you expect to be (a) stronger and more agile, (b) the same, or (c) weaker and less agile than you are today?"

■ "If you expect to remain the same or improve, list three things you do daily to ensure that outcome." (Remind them of the research documenting gradual decline.)

■ "If you think significant decline is unavoidable, is that expectation based on personal beliefs, media images, misconceptions, or norms?" (Share new research.)

■ "Are you satisfied with the expected outcome?"

■ "If not, what are you willing to do to prevent a negative outcome"?

Opportunity

To reach a broad range of people, we must make opportunities available within each dimension of wellness, at multiple levels of functional ability,

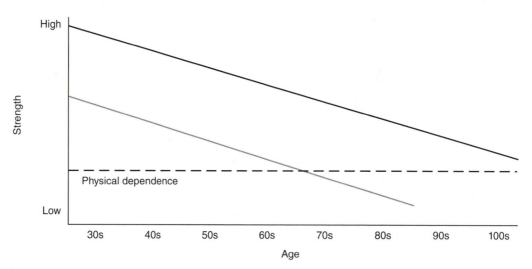

▶ **Figure 3.2** Relationship between strength and functional independence.

and through each stage of behavior change. Refer to chapter 1 (pp. 8-13) for more information on the six dimensions of wellness and chapter 4 (pp. 53-55) for more information on levels of functional ability. The sidebar on page 33 outlines the stages of change and offers ideas for meeting the needs of people at each stage of change.

Opportunities for resistance training can include making resistance bands, ankle weights, and handheld weights easily available to potential clients along with simple function-based exercise brochures and exercise videos or DVDs with easy-to-follow instructions. Self-directed resources can reach people in the action stage of change and can encourage people in contemplation and preparation stages, who may be reluctant to join a group exercise program, to move into action.

For example, wellness stations (see figure 3.1, p. 36) and simple function-based exercises (see figure 3.3) that can be posted on bulletin boards or placed in newsletters offer ongoing, easy access to opportunities that do not require people to take a specific action (i.e., go out of their way) to engage. These types of resources reach everyone but are especially effective for reaching people who are in precontemplation, contemplation, and preparation.

Activity of the Week

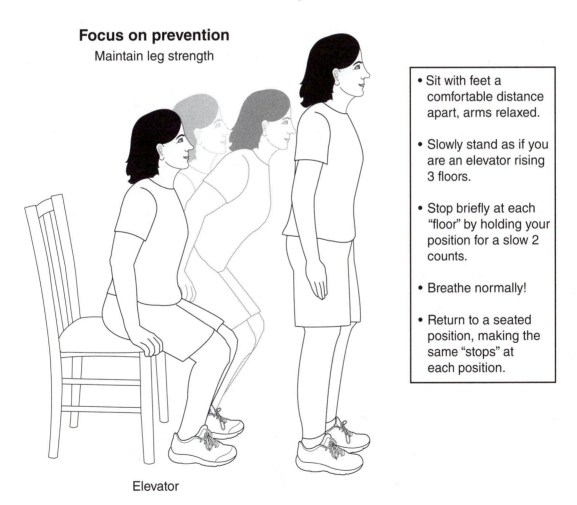

Focus on prevention

Maintain leg strength

- Sit with feet a comfortable distance apart, arms relaxed.

- Slowly stand as if you are an elevator rising 3 floors.

- Stop briefly at each "floor" by holding your position for a slow 2 counts.

- Breathe normally!

- Return to a seated position, making the same "stops" at each position.

Elevator

Leg strength helps prevent falls

▶ **Figure 3.3** Simple, function-based exercise that can be posted for easy access.

© Kay Van Norman.

Resistance training classes, on the other hand, are good for reaching people in the action or maintenance stages. When creating self-directed resources, use simple exercises that focus on basic functional tasks like rising from a chair, climbing stairs, walking, and dressing. Visit www.kayvannorman.com for Project MOVE resources.

Additional strategies include offering periodic, short workshops on different kinds of movement classes so clients can try out an activity without any implied commitment. Movement breaks throughout the day, like 5-minute movement sessions right before meals, also invite participation without any implied commitment to a regular class, which is often important for people in the first three stages of change.

Verification

Verification refers to the ongoing access to information and opportunities. It uses the multiple contact points developed for *opportunity* to reinforce or verify that a person is making the right decision to begin resistance training or at the very least should consider it as a viable strategy to improve functional ability. Verification reinforces information presented in seminars and classes. It encourages ongoing discussion about the topic and normalizes the idea that resistance training is safe and effective for almost all people.

Table tents with fast facts about strength, power, and function and bulletin boards that address resistance training with specific ideas for engagement are effective verification strategies. Weekly newsletters or other correspondence can reinforce the messages through articles, personal testimonials, and basic functional exercises and provide ongoing invitations for involvement. In addition to providing ongoing verification of the benefit of strength training, look for ways to encourage self-responsibility and a positive attitude toward improving well-being. One example is seen in figure 3.1 (p. 36). A person may walk past the station multiple times and only read the banner statement or look at the artwork. Some may stop and read the positive affirmation statement. Perhaps the tenth time they walk by the station they will engage in the physical activity component. Regardless of how much they chose to engage, the message of self-responsibility for well-being is always clear.

Pre- and postprogram assessments to measure basic functional ability and track improvement in leg strength and power, balance, and arm strength and power are an important part of the verification element. Link positive changes with personally relevant activities such as the ability to lift and play with grandchildren, carry a suitcase, and perform other independent living tasks. The Senior Fitness Test (Rikli and Jones, 2001) is a simple, well-documented assessment that can be used to track and verify progress.

Education

The education component includes providing clients and potential clients with practical application research documenting the link between resistance training and functional independence. Research by Fiatarone (1994) offers a dramatic demonstration of how strength training is safe and effective for almost everyone. Her study of nursing home residents aged 72 to 98 with multiple chronic conditions demonstrated significant gains in strength (113%) and improved function. Its inclusion of advanced-age and physically impaired subjects and findings of injury rates lower than the average for all age groups make this study personally relevant to many adults older than 65 with chronic conditions or physical impairments. In addition, a review of power training research done by Hazell and colleagues (2007) demonstrates the critical link between power and function (see figure 1.4, chapter 1).

Refute old research that claimed older adults cannot improve strength and power, and offer new research showing that misguided protocols, *not aging*, resulted in the misconception that loss of function is an unavoidable consequence of aging. Making the research personally relevant helps clients recognize where they are on the scale of functional independence. Use functional assessments and encourage clients to assess their perceived well-being to evaluate whether they are doing what they can to maximize strength, power, and function to retain independence. Refer to chapter 7 for an explanation of how to integrate these concepts into programming in senior-living communities.

WELLNESS WRAP-UP

Psychosocial aspects of aging and physical activity can create motives for and barriers to participation in physical activity and other wellness programs. Perceptions of self and perceptions of aging and physical activity affect motivation and compliance and determine whether a person is open to the message of whole-person wellness. Understanding psychosocial concepts will help you integrate multiple dimensions of wellness into each program offering and identify triggers and barriers to participation. It will also help you identify strategies that will appeal to clients at each level of functional ability and each stage of change.

The MOVE approach ensures that you provide clients with ongoing motivation, opportunities, verification, and education. It is a great way to integrate psychosocial concepts to create well-rounded programs.

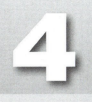

Programming Guidelines

Meeting the needs of class participants who have different levels of functional ability and health status and who are in various stages of change requires attention to many details. This chapter provides practical strategies to help you create the optimal environment for learning and addresses safety issues in programming. It outlines how to develop a well-rounded program with quality instruction and good class management procedures. The chapter also reinforces the need to use a whole-person wellness approach and offers strategies to support the psychosocial components of well-being. Finally, this chapter discusses the main components of a fitness class, including the warm-up and cool-down, aerobic conditioning, flexibility, strength and power, and coordination and balance.

PROGRAM COMPONENTS

Several important components form the foundation of any class—the instructor, the schedule, the class format, and the music. Paying attention to these elements will help you build a program that meets the needs of your target population.

Instructor Qualities

One of the most important elements of any exercise program is the instructor. Exercise leaders must give safety a high priority and be able to match programming to functional abilities. At the very least, instructors need certifications in cardiopulmonary resuscitation (CPR) and first aid. Additional certifications, such as lifeguard or emergency water safety, are required for water exercise if the pool does not have a lifeguard on duty during class time.

It is best to have a physical education or health-related background, which provides a depth of knowledge concerning the body's response to exercise. However, if you do not have a formal education in this area, a reputable exercise instructor certification program can provide the information you need to create quality programs. A good certification program will help you understand the major muscle groups and which ones are responsible for creating specific movements. The certification program should ensure that you understand how to program at the proper intensity and should offer guidelines for improving cardiovascular endurance, strength, flexibility, balance, and coordination. It should also offer basic first aid and CPR training and thoroughly cover safety and liability issues for instructors. Commit to continuing education after completing a certification to ensure that you

develop a practical understanding of all elements of programming. If the information is new to you, talk to a physical education professional, a physical therapist, or some other health professional who deals with the movement of the body. Study your resources, and then ask these movement professionals specific questions to determine whether your understanding is correct.

Senior exercise certifications have become an industry standard for instructors who lead classes of older adults, even for those with physical education and health-related backgrounds. These certifications offer extensive information on special conditions and circumstances relevant to senior exercise instruction. National standards for preparing senior fitness instructors in the United States were first published in the *Journal of Aging and Physical Activity* (Jones and Clark, 1998). More recently, Jones and Rose (2005) included updated standards in the appendix of *Physical Activity Instruction of Older Adults*. Also see the International Society for Aging and Physical Activity's Web site (www.isapa.org/guidelines/index.cfm) for a free download of complete international standards, now titled "International Curriculum Guidelines for Preparing Physical Activity Instructors of Older Adults." Other sources of physical activity guidelines for older adults include the American College of Sports Medicine's *Guidelines for Exercise Testing and Prescription* (8th edition) and guidelines from the U.S. Centers for Disease Control and Prevention (www.cdc.gov/physicalactivity/everyone/guidelines/olderadults.html). Quality training programs for senior exercise instructors should meet these standards. Some certifications focus only on physically independent and physically fit adults, whereas others provide education on working with adults of all functional abilities. Only consider certifications from reputable organizations. Many companies selling certifications in older adult exercise are not legitimate, and quick online senior exercise certifications simply do not offer enough information to be of value. Refer to the following list of reputable organizations providing exercise certifications and education in older adult exercise.

- Administration on Aging: www.aoa.gov
- Aerobic and Fitness Association of America: www.afaa.com
- American College of Sports Medicine: www.acsm.org
- American Council on Exercise: www.acefitness.org

- American Fitness Professionals & Associates: www.afpafitness.com
- American Senor Fitness Association: www.seniorfitness.net
- American Society on Aging: www.asaging.org
- Canadian Fitness Professionals: www.canfitpro.com
- Cooper Institute: www.cooperinstitute.org
- DSW Fitness: www.dswfitness.com
- International Council on Active Aging: www.icaa.cc
- National Council on Aging: www.ncoa.org
- Provincial Fitness Unit of Alberta: www.provincialfitnessunit.ca

Some students will rely heavily on their exercise instructor as a health resource. Be well informed on the latest information in exercise and other health-related areas but do not step past the bounds of your knowledge. It is not unusual for class participants to ask you to confirm or refute their doctors' advice in a variety of areas. Contradicting a doctor's advice poses an unacceptable safety and liability risk. See page 51 for more information on liability issues.

A health history questionnaire will inform you about any special physical needs of participants, but it is also important to get to know the participants in your program. Consciously create a class with a personal environment. Most successful programs demonstrate instructor–student relationships that go beyond just being friendly and upbeat to getting to know each other as people, including family and personal interests.

Show up 15 minutes early for class, and you may notice that it becomes the norm for others to arrive early to warm up and visit with others. This is an excellent time to learn about participants. Allow 5 to 10 minutes to answer questions or just interact after class. Contact students who suddenly stop attending to see whether they are well. Most people will appreciate a call to check on their well-being and will be pleased to note that they were missed.

Create an environment that helps participants get to know and interact with each other as well. Providing social interaction during class time will

Motivating Instructors

I took a few days going from class to class to ask the students what qualities they like to see in an exercise instructor. "Enthusiasm," June says. ""Yes," Alice agrees. "We need someone who can motivate us to move by making class fun. The instructor also must be willing to do the exercises with us because in the pool it is difficult to hear instructions; many times we just follow with what the instructor is doing on the pool deck."

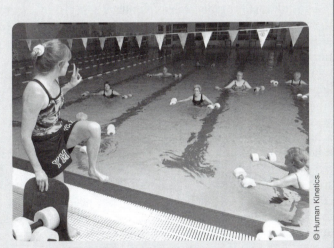
© Human Kinetics.

"They need to perform the exercises in the right order," Minnie says, "starting slowly and working up to the more difficult aerobics, and then giving a good cool-down."

"I like it when instructors walk around the pool area and watch each person," June adds. "Then you know they care if you are doing the exercises properly."

Enthusiasm and being fun to exercise with also rank high in the low-impact aerobics class. "I like an instructor who can get me motivated on those days that I have a hard time getting up and getting to class," Elsie says. "When the instructor is enthusiastic it makes me glad I made the effort to get here, and when class is over I know the day's off to a good start."

"I appreciate an instructor who uses good music and keeps rhythm with the music," Norma says.

"And someone who keeps us moving and gives us a good workout," Bob adds.

They all agree wholeheartedly: As long as they are putting in the time, they like to get a good workout!

encourage students to develop a new network of friends who might become part of their daily lives. This more personal atmosphere between instructor and student, and between student and student, gradually creates a bond of trust and respect within the class and becomes an important reason why people attend.

Class Organization

Quality instruction must be paired with good class organization and management skills. Class scheduling and location can affect how many people will try the class. Once people attend, then the format, music, and general atmosphere of the class will largely determine whether they continue. Each of these factors can significantly influence the success of an exercise program, so they must be carefully planned.

Scheduling Considerations

The hours of 8, 9, and 10 in the morning are very popular for adult exercise classes. Midafternoon can also be popular. Because these hours are nonpeak hours in most fitness clubs, these facilities have an added incentive to develop adult programs. During summer months the Bozeman, Montana–based Young at Heart Program offers a popular 7 a.m. class to accommodate participants' busy summer schedules. The specific hour scheduled is less important than consistency: Clubs should offer a consistent schedule from week to week. Do not assume that any time is satisfactory simply because many mature adults are retired from formal employment. A consistent weekly schedule allows participants to form a habit of exercise class that fits into their other scheduled responsibilities.

Always hold the class in the same location. Most students like to get comfortable in familiar surroundings, so a class that bounces from one place to the next may not have good attendance. Exercising at one location also allows effective use of bulletin boards or other information centers. Stopping at a bulletin board that provides health information, wellness opportunities in the community, thoughts for the day, and schedule updates will soon become a regular part of the class members' routine.

Class Format

There are several effective class formats. The standard 1-hour format with 10 to 20 minutes of warm-up, 20 to 30 minutes of aerobics, and 15 to 20 minutes of cool-down and stretching works well (refer to chapter 5 for specific exercises). Classes for beginners will have longer phases for the warm-up and the cool-down and stretching. As participants become more fit you may increase the time spent doing aerobics, and some of the warm-ups can approach low-level aerobics. Always, however, maintain at least 10 minutes of warm-up and 15 minutes of cool-down and stretching. Allowing students to perform aerobic exercise without proper warm-up and cool-down can pose health risks for them and liability risks for your program.

If you have access to strength training machines and cardiovascular exercise equipment (e.g., stationary bikes, steppers), consider a 90-minute "stations" format. For example, offer a 30-minute warm-up of the participants' choice (stationary bike, walking, light strength training), followed by 30 minutes of aerobics of the participants' choice (water or low-impact exercise, stair climber, stationary bike) and then 30 minutes of cool-down and stretching (tai chi, yoga, floor work, water-based stretching). When using this type of format you must carefully explain the required phases (warm-up, aerobics, cool-down) and monitor individual progress to ensure that students are achieving the proper balance. This format also poses challenges in maintaining the social aspect, especially group cohesion. You may want to do at least one phase of the class, such as the cool-down, as a group. As you develop flexible programs that make use of the equipment available to you, also take the time to plan forums for social interaction.

The warm-up and cool-down phases of class lend themselves well to social interaction. This social component is of vital importance to classes and a strong motivator for people of all ages to continue to attend class. Designate class time for interaction, and structure instruction to promote interaction. Warm-ups or cool-downs done in a circle and in partners will facilitate conversation. Maintain a friendly banter throughout the class so all participants will feel free to talk. If possible create a space where students can come early or stay late to interact, have a beverage, and generally feel at home and part of something special.

Music

Music plays a significant role in the success of an exercise class, so be sure the music you choose contributes to participants' overall enjoyment. The music should be generation appropriate, that is, music that participants can relate to and feel comfortable with. Imagine walking into an aerobics class filled with college students and using music from the 1940s for the entire class. The idea of using only current Top 40 hits in a class for mature adults is just

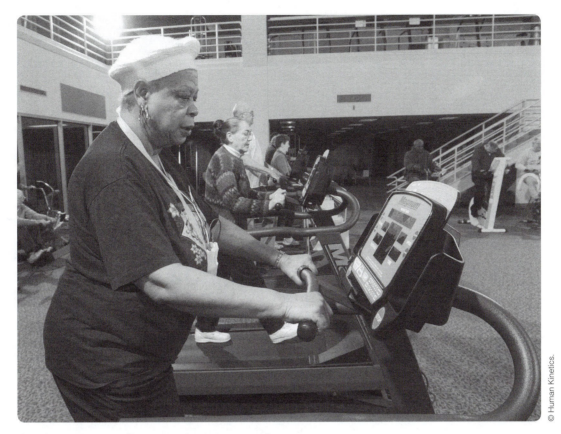

© Human Kinetics.

Cardio machines offer a good warm-up option.

as ridiculous, and it will yield the same results—an unenthusiastic group today and an empty room next session. When you use music that is popular with participants, they will sing along, reminisce, and truly enjoy their time in class.

However, don't restrict music selections only to "oldies" tunes; popular songs can be used as well. Try playing new songs between oldies and watch reactions. Then ask participants which songs they liked. Look for songs that are pleasant to listen to or sing along with and are fun and upbeat for aerobics or slow and relaxing for cool-down. Use music that you also enjoy, because this will promote your own enthusiasm. Refer to the sidebar for a list of music that has been consistently well received in the classes I've taught.

Choose music that has a distinct rhythm without overpowering vocals; midrange vocals with simple instrumental accompaniment and clearly understood words work well. Instrumentals with a distinct continuous rhythm are another good choice, but avoid those with excessive embellishment of the melody—the rhythm may get lost in embellishment and become difficult for participants to follow.

Consider the appropriate volume of the music. The potential for students with hearing difficulties increases in older adult classes. Some hearing impairments will be partially corrected by hearing aids, but others will be completely uncorrected. This does not mean you should turn the music up louder! Many people dislike loud music, and those who have some degree of hearing loss will not necessarily benefit from the increased volume. In most cases, they will strain to hear your instructions, and loud music will only make this more difficult. Students with hearing aids will be most troubled by loud music because the aid magnifies all sounds, which produces an uncomfortable and irritating jumble of music, voices, and background noises. For people with hearing impairment who wear hearing aids, music with very high-pitched instrumental or vocal notes can be very uncomfortable. Play music at a modest volume and notice how students respond to the music. Ask them whether they can hear the rhythm and whether they would like an adjustment in the volume. It won't be long before you can easily recognize the appropriate volume for each class.

EXAMPLES OF MUSIC

The following songs are appropriate for the warm-up and cool-down phases:

▶ Max Bygraves: midrange vocals for warm-up and cool-down
▶ Glenn Miller: big band vocal and instrumental selections for warm-up and cool-down
▶ John Denver: midrange vocals for warm-up and cool-down
▶ George Winston: nice instrumental piano selections for cool-down and relaxation
▶ Mark Knopfler: *Princess Bride* soundtrack; instrumental relaxation
▶ Ray Lynch: nice instrumentals for warm-ups, especially "Deep Breakfast" and "Celestial Soda Pop"

These songs are appropriate for aerobics:

▶ Max Bygraves: midrange vocals, many in three- or four-song medleys such as "Won't You Come Home Bill Bailey?" and "Bye, Bye Blackbird" (available for ordering; check with music stores or online)
▶ Herb Alpert: many moderate-tempo instrumental selections, like "Spanish Flea," "Sentimental Over You"
▶ Glenn Miller: many moderate-tempo selections, vocal and instrumental, like "In the Mood," "Chattanooga Choo Choo"
▶ Roger Miller: midrange vocals, like "Engine Number 9," "England Swings," "King of the Road"
▶ Broadway show tunes, such as "Hello Dolly" and "Cabaret"
▶ Royal Philharmonic Orchestra instrumental medleys, like "Hooked on Classics" I, II, and III
▶ Manhattan Swing Orchestra instrumental medleys, like "Hooked on Swing"

SAFETY

Safety is a high priority in an exercise class designed for older adults. Age is a risk factor for numerous chronic conditions that significantly affect exercise safety, including coronary artery disease, high blood pressure, heart disease, osteoporosis, arthritis, and muscle and joint dysfunction. People who have been sedentary before beginning an exercise class run a higher risk for heart attacks, strokes, joint and muscle injuries, and fractures. Sedentary adults may also exhibit significant deficits in balance, coordination, and strength that can pose a high risk of falling. Sensory impairments such as low vision or hearing and medications that affect depth perception and reaction time can add to exercise risk.

To manage these risks, apply your foundational knowledge of exercise science and levels of functional ability to all aspects of the exercise class and create programs that are as safe as possible even for participants with undiagnosed conditions such as heart disease, osteoporosis, and balance abnormalities. Provide a thorough warm-up, carefully monitor aerobic exercise intensity, and ensure a proper cool-down to allow participants adequate time to recover from the aerobic phase before they leave class. When creating movement patterns, weigh the risks against the benefits of all movement choices to enhance safety for exercisers across the range of functional abilities. Designing the warm-up and cool-down, monitoring intensity, and choosing safe movements are discussed in more detail later in the chapter. An excellent resource for detailed modifications appropriate to numerous chronic conditions is *ACSM's Exercise Management for Persons With Chronic Diseases and Disabilities* (Durstine and Moore, 2003).

Environmental Risks

Be aware of any environmental hazards in the facility in which the class is held. For example, a hot room is unsafe for aerobic conditioning. Those with high blood pressure are at greater risk of cardiac problems when they become overheated. If participants become red faced, perspire significantly, or mention how hot the room feels, it is too hot! Be sensitive to how your own body is responding to exercise; this will alert you to signs of excessive heat in your students. If the room cannot be better ventilated or the room temperature lowered, do not attempt aerobic conditioning.

In contrast, a room that is too cool will make it difficult to adequately warm up before aerobic movement. Many adults who have been sedentary have reduced flexibility of the muscles, tendons, and ligaments, increasing their risk of muscle pulls and strains. A cold room can significantly reduce these participants' ability to warm up (i.e., increase core temperature). A room is too cold if you or your students feel chilled during the warm-up and experience an uncomfortably rapid cool-down after the aerobic phase. It is very difficult to provide a proper (i.e., gradual) cool-down and safe stretching for participants in a cold room. Pay attention to the exercise surface. Look for slick, sticky, or uneven spots on the floor. A fall or trip can mean embarrassment and bruises to some exercisers or a possibly life-threatening fracture to adults with conditions such as osteoporosis. See chapter 7 for information on finding appropriate environments for adult exercise programs.

Minimizing Liability

Liability is a topic of concern for any exercise class, but it is of special concern when you work with high-risk participants. For your protection and the protection of your participants, require them to consult with a physician before starting your exercise program. Basic health information will make you aware of health issues that could affect exercise safety. A functional assessment will identify issues that could place the client at risk because of muscle weakness, balance deficits, or an extremely low level of aerobic endurance. An informed consent form (see figure 4.1) should ask specific questions about high blood pressure, heart disease, diabetes, coronary artery disease, osteoporosis, arthritis, asthma, any cardiorespiratory abnormalities, and medications used. Many people will neglect to include important information unless it is specifically requested. Be aware that even a signed informed consent form will not protect you from a lawsuit if you act in a negligent manner. Allen (2005) provides an excellent overview of legal issues related to teaching adult exercise classes, including risk management, medical emergency prevention and response, facility standards, and accepted standards of instruction and care.

Interview new participants concerning their past and present activity levels. Perform a simple functional assessment to determine basic levels of upper- and lower-body strength and mobility, dynamic balance, and aerobic endurance. Refer to the *Senior Fitness Test Manual* by Rikli and Jones (2001) for a simple, well-documented functional assessment. These strategies will help you make informed recommendations about the type and duration of exercise in which participants can safely participate. These strategies will also make participants aware of the importance of proper exercise intensity and encourage them to set specific goals. Update the screening information yearly to stay informed of any changes in a participant's health status, and repeat assessments periodically to gauge progress.

Emergency Procedures

A well-rehearsed emergency plan is essential. This plan must involve all of the steps necessary to care for an injured or ill person and to summon medical help. In the case of an emergency during class, it is likely that a class participant will call for emergency personnel while you provide care to the injured party. Post all emergency procedures next to the telephone using large, high-contrast, easily readable print (e.g., black print on white paper). Readability is even more critical for water-exercise classes in which participants may not be wearing corrective lenses.

Each instructor should have a list of the students in class, including information on any participant who has a high-risk medical condition (this information is taken from the screening forms). This will help the instructor and emergency personnel deal effectively with the situation. Privacy laws require that personal medical information be kept confidential, so consider using a coding system on roll sheets and keep them in your possession.

Rehearse all emergency procedures with your classes on a regular basis so that everyone involved is confident of the procedures. Participants are well aware of the possibility of illness or injury during exercise and will be more comfortable knowing there is a solid, workable plan for such emergencies. Keep written records of any health incident or accident occurring in class, including the date and

Name of physician _____ Phone _____

Person to notify in emergency _____

Relationship_____ Phone _____

You may contact my physician if necessary   Y_____ N _____

I am aware of having the following condition(s):

       Heart disease _____ High blood pressure _____ Diabetes_____

       Lung disease _____ Cancer _____ Osteoporosis _____

       Peripheral vascular disease_____ Neurological condition_____

       Balance abnormality _____ Other_____

I am currently on the following medication that regulates my heart rate: _____

_____ None _____

I am currently on these additional medications: _____

_____

_____

_____

PLEASE READ

The Young at Heart program involves exercises to develop muscle strength, power, and endurance, aerobic capacity, flexibility, balance, and coordination. Although each participant is encouraged to proceed at his or her own pace, as with all exercise some risk of injury is present. For this reason, a physician's consultation is required before participation in the program.

RELEASE

I, the undersigned, have discussed Young at Heart with my physician and, being mindful of my age, health, physical condition, and medical status, am voluntarily participating in the Young at Heart exercise program. Therefore, I hereby release Young at Heart, its representatives, and their successors from liability for accident, injury, or illness that I may incur as a result of participation in the program, and I hereby assume these risks.

_____   _____

Date   Signature of participant

▶ **Figure 4.1** Sample liability form.

From K. Van Norman, 2010, *Exercise and wellness for older adults*, 2nd ed. (Champaign, IL: Human Kinetics).

time of the incident, name and address of injured party, suspected cause of injury, detailed description of injury or illness, detailed description of how the instructor responded to the incident, what actions were taken (e.g., participant was sent to hospital, released to a friend, went home), and anything else that could help you recall specifics at a later date.

WELL-ROUNDED PROGRAMS

A well-rounded program will focus on the functional level of participants and their most immediate needs. Program designers must provide safe movements by weighing the benefits against the potential risks for movement choices. Finally, the program must meet more than just physical needs; it should actively support emotional and social elements of well-being.

Levels of Function and Needs

It is imperative to identify the current levels of functional ability within your class. In *Physical Dimensions of Aging* (2005), Spirduso identifies five distinct levels of function: physically dependent, physically frail, physically independent, physically fit, and physically elite.

Using this five-level concept, I have identified priority needs for each group and suggested movement choices (see table 4.1). Although aerobic conditioning is very beneficial, it is not the highest priority for those within the first two levels of function, who struggle to perform the most basic activities of daily living. Programming to meet participants' most immediate needs ensures that they can be successful in movement and offers them the best opportunity to move from one level to the next. Function-based activity for physically dependent and frail people can also result in small improvements in cardiovascular function. Please refer to chapter 5 for specific exercises appropriate to each level.

When creating programs for physically dependent and physically frail participants, focus on movement that improves physical function for basic self-care. These people need the strength, power, mobility, balance, and coordination necessary for self-feeding, bathing, dressing, using the toilet, transferring, and walking. Focus on finger and hand strength and mobility, arm strength, shoulder and hip range of motion, leg strength and power, ankle strength and range of motion, and foot and toe mobility.

Evaluate the specific movements necessary to accomplish a functional task and build your program around them. For example, using the toilet requires enough strength in the hips, knees, and ankles to go from a standing to a seated position and back to standing. It also requires enough strength and mobility in the legs, hips, hands, and arms to remove and replace clothing. Wheelchair-bound people require enough upper-body strength to transfer from the chair to the toilet and back. Refer to table 4.1 for levels of function, needs, and recommended activities.

Safe Movements

Group classes will have participants with a range of functional abilities, and those with diminished levels of strength, balance, or coordination (conditions that in some cases are exacerbated by sensory impairments) are at risk for falling. Statistics also show that some degree of osteopenia (bone thinning) is common in older women, placing them at high risk for fractures. Therefore, in land-based aerobic programs, activities that require quick footwork with surprise changes of direction could cause ankle turns, trips, and falls and do not meet the basic standard of safety (benefits vs. risks).

Carefully weigh the potential risks against the benefits of each type of exercise or movement. Choose smooth rather than jerky movements and completed movements rather than choppy or jerky starts and stops. Use low-impact movements that keep at least one foot in contact with the floor at all times, coupled with simple movement patterns. Smooth, completed movements reduce the risk of joint stress and injury to participants. In land-based exercise classes, low-impact movements are the most appropriate choice for adults. High-impact movements pose a significantly higher risk of injury for all ages with minimal potential for increased results. Smooth, controlled movements and low-impact activities offer the same benefits for strength, range of motion, and endurance without stressing the joints and muscles. See chapter 5 for examples of safe, effective movement sequences.

In addition to being safer, simple movements and movement combinations promote self-confidence and self-efficacy by promoting success in movement. Many adults have lost some degree of coordination if they have not been regularly participating in activities requiring coordination. For this reason, rapid changes of direction and complicated movement patterns increase both participant anxiety and the danger of falling. Such activities can also decrease

Table 4.1   Levels of Function, Needs, and Sample Activities

Level of function	Needs	Recommended activities
Physically dependent: cannot execute some or all of the BADLs Are dependent on others for basic functions of living	Strength, range of motion, balance, and coordination necessary for basic self-care (BADLs): • Self-feeding • Bathing • Dressing • Toileting • Transferring • Walking ROM and strength in the hips, knees, legs, ankles, shoulders, arms, wrists, and hands Speed of movement Ankle flexion, foot mobility, and hand and finger mobility	• Chair and chair-assisted exercise addressing the BADLs • One-on-one water-based exercise • One-on-one strength and power training • Function-based exercise for upper and lower body • Seated coordination activities • Seated speed of movement activities with special focus on ankle, hand, and finger strength and mobility • One-on-one balance training • One-on-one gait training • Physical and occupational therapy • Seated recreational activities • Breathing and relaxation • Seated ball toss, stamping bugs
Physically frail: can perform the BADLs but cannot perform some or all of the activities necessary to live independently May have a debilitating disease or condition that physically challenges them daily	Muscular strength, power, and endurance; low-level cardiovascular endurance; ROM; balance; coordination necessary to perform BADLs and IADLs (e.g., meal preparation, shopping) Note to instructor: Use same exercises for physically dependent people and include additional activities challenging balance and addressing postural and gait abnormalities.	Any of exercises listed for physically dependent people plus the following: • Group water-based programming (e.g., water walking) • Modified tai chi and yoga • Supervised group strength and power training • Modified recreational games • Seated dance activities • Chair exercise with 5-minute segments of aerobic endurance • Walking
Physically independent: live independently, usually without debilitating symptoms of major chronic diseases May have low health and fitness reserves May function very close to maximum capacity just to live independently	Muscular strength, endurance, and flexibility; joint ROM; balance; coordination; and cardiovascular endurance exercise to remain physically independent and prevent illness, disability, and injury Education on the importance of prevention of functional loss; encouragement to increase health and fitness reserves Note to instructor: Take into account the range of functional ability within this level. Some are close to being fit and many are at risk for becoming frail due to inactivity.	Any of the activities listed above plus these: • Chair aerobics • Low-impact aerobics • Line, folk, social dancing • Water aerobics • Lap swimming • Walking courses • Tai chi and yoga • Circuit training • Strength and power training • Recreational and sports activities
Physically fit: exercise at least two times a week for their health, enjoyment, and well-being Generally are very physically active either in a job or recreational activities Have high health and fitness reserves	Muscular strength, power, and endurance; joint ROM; balance; coordination; agility; and cardiovascular endurance Information on injury prevention and recovery Variety of opportunities to maintain level of fitness Education on appropriate exercise intensity and injury prevention and treatment.	All activities

Level of function	Needs	Recommended activities
Physically elite: train almost daily May compete in sports, work in a physically demanding job, or participate in strenuous recreational activities Usually very motivated to stay active; enjoy very high health and fitness reserves	Programming for muscular strength, power, and endurance; flexibility and agility; and high levels of cardiovascular endurance Injury prevention and recovery Activity-specific training to improve performance in a desired area Notes to instructor: Help these participants maintain their level of fitness and provide conditioning for improving performance in competition or in strenuous activities. Your primary role with physically elite adults is to be a facilitator.	All activities

BADLs = basic activities of daily living; ROM = range of motion; IADLs = independent activities of daily living.

self-esteem and enjoyment for those who are unsuccessful in executing the movement. See chapter 3 for a discussion of the importance of programming to improve self-esteem and self-efficacy.

The need for simple movement poses an extra challenge for you to come up with an interesting variety of movement combinations, music, and teaching formations. Vary the basic front-facing formation by using circles, lines, and partner groupings. Such varied formations add interest and facilitate social interaction. Many folk dances can be modified to meet safety guidelines and add a great deal of fun and social interaction to classes. See chapter 5 for specific exercises and movement patterns.

Psychosocial Components

The emotional and social components of an adult exercise program contribute significantly to its success. Even programs that successfully meet the

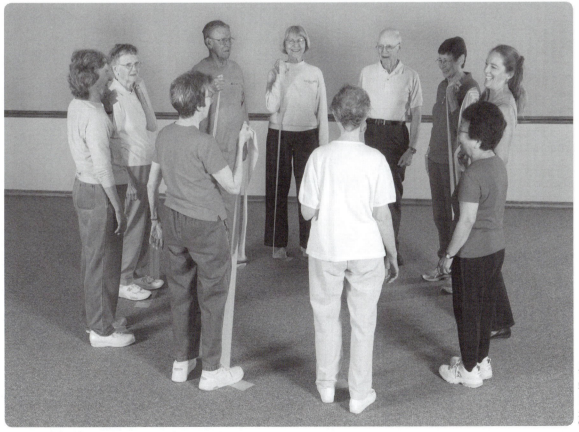

Exercise classes provide a support network.

© Human Kinetics.

exercise needs of participants can stagnate if participants' emotional well-being and social interaction are not addressed. On the other hand, programs that focus on emotional well-being and social interaction, even if they lack some important exercise components, gather more participants despite the deficiencies. The instructor determines the atmosphere of the class and is ultimately responsible for supporting multiple dimensions of well-being. Refer to chapter 1 for more information about the six dimensions of wellness and to chapter 3 for a discussion of psychosocial concepts related to adult exercise programming.

Social Interaction

Social contact with others is consistently one of the top five answers to the question I ask in my program, "Why do you come to this exercise class?" Most participants look forward to exercise class as an important part of their day. It is a place to meet others with similar interests and be a significant part of a group. For example, people who have lost spouses often find themselves among longtime friends who are still couples and can feel like third wheels at social gatherings. Members of an exercise group can become a unique support system for each other. Carpooling to class, taking part in activities before or after class, and socializing outside of class all help expand the exercise participant's support network. In addition, regular participants know that if they don't show up for class, others will ask about them and likely call to check on them. For participants who live alone, knowing that others are watching out for them is a tremendous benefit of being a regular part of an exercise group.

Devote some time in each class to social interaction, and actively facilitate participant interaction throughout the class. See chapters 5 and 6 for ideas and activities. When the students become comfortable as a group, an activity such as the shoulder circle rub (p. 99 in chapter 5) is an effective way to facilitate talking and laughing—and it feels great!

Classes Offer Social Connections

By 6:30 a.m., the early-morning water exercisers are dressed and ready a good half hour before their class and are sitting on the benches talking and laughing. Many in this group have been attending the same early-morning class for 6 years.

Asked the standard question about what keeps them coming to water exercise, Minnie says, "Arthritis. If I weren't exercising, I would barely be able to move." "It just makes me feel good," says Anne. The others agree. When asked why they get here so early, they look at each other and chuckle. "It's easier to find a parking place if you get here early," June says. They come up with other sensible reasons, such as not liking to hurry to get dressed and allowing plenty of time in case they have

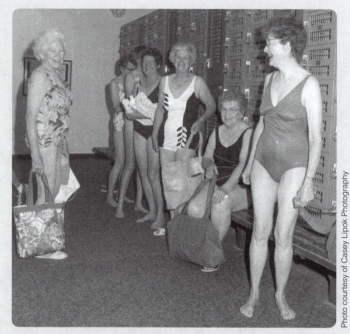

Photo courtesy of Casey Lipok Photography

car problems. Then Mary says, "When you have exercised with the same people for 5 to 6 years, you get kind of attached to them." Helen laughs and adds, "We have lots of visiting to get done, and you can't do that in class while you're concentrating on the exercises." The smiles and nods confirm that this social interaction with people they have grown to care about is the real reason these participants can be found perched on the benches in the locker room long before class begins.

Emotional Well-Being

A positive, noncompetitive environment with many opportunities for enjoyment and success in movement will help support the emotional well-being of participants. Make a special effort to ensure that all participants can be successful movers in your class. All participants want to believe they can successfully perform the exercises and exercise combinations in a class, and those who are less confident in movement can experience anxiety. Many participants may not have exercised in a group setting for many years, possibly since elementary school. They may come into class worrying that they can't keep up. If your class approach and content reinforce that idea, these people will take this as a confirmation that they are not capable of exercise. Your job is to make sure participants are successful in movement the majority of the time.

Avoid complex combinations and complicated steps. Use simple movement patterns and easy-to-follow rhythmic patterns. Provide a noncompetitive environment in which all are encouraged to work at their own levels, and frequently demonstrate variations appropriate to different levels of ability. Give positive reinforcement for all accomplishments and efforts, and make adjustments when you see students struggling.

A highly effective teaching technique is to have a simple "home-base" step, such as marching in place, which everyone can perform easily and return to frequently. A home-base step before and after a new movement gives each participant a chance to be successful a large percentage of the time and provides a positive exercise experience. Face the class when performing a new combination (mirroring movements) to observe how well participants are doing, and frequently return to the home-base step when necessary. Feeling at ease in performing movement to music will increase the participants' self-esteem and promote a feeling of accomplishment.

Once participants feel successful, you can present additional challenges like more complex patterns interspersed with the simple home-base movement. Challenges met with success further increase self-esteem and self-efficacy and encourage confidence when people face other challenges, not only in exercise but in other areas of life. Always balance challenge with ensured success, and always weigh the benefits against the potential risks for all movements. Refer to chapter 3 for detailed information about psychosocial aspects of aging and how they affect motivation and compliance in exercise and wellness programming, and see chapter 5 for specific movement sequences.

COMPONENTS OF A FITNESS CLASS

An exercise class should include a warm-up and cool-down and as many of the other components of fitness as possible, including well-planned and monitored aerobic conditioning, techniques to promote strength and power, and activities to improve flexibility, coordination, and balance. Of course some classes will be more specialized, like a strength and power training class, but regardless of the main exercise component the body needs an opportunity to warmup and cooldown.

Importance of Warming Up and Cooling Down

Warm-up and cool-down exercises are designed to provide a safe transition into, and an adequate recovery from, more vigorous exercise. Proper warm-up and cool-down phases are an important safety precaution for managing exercise risks. They are also a great time to establish social and emotional connections between you and the class and between participants. Use a circle formation during parts of the warm-up to allow close contact between participants and opportunities for friendly exchanges. Teach simple social mixer dances and activities during the warm-up to help participants learn each other's names and ensure that everyone is involved in the social interactions.

Designate time during the warm-up and cool-down to converse with students and encourage interaction. Use 3 to 5 minutes at the beginning of the warm-up to define goals for class time and ask students to think of one goal for themselves. For example, an instructor's goal may be to have students perform a simple coordination sequence they already know to a slightly faster tempo, and a student's goal may be to stretch further on a particular exercise. This approach at the beginning of class prompts participants to engage in mindful exercise.

Warming Up

The purpose of warming up is to increase the body temperature and provide a gradual transition into more vigorous exercise. Proper warm-up reduces the risk of musculoskeletal injury and increases efficiency of both the neuromuscular system and aerobic metabolism. It should also set the stage for safe and effective exercise by establishing proper movement techniques and reinforcing techniques for monitoring exercise intensity. Finally, the warm-up should engage class participants socially, emotionally, and cognitively.

An active warm-up (using body movements to increase the body temperature) is preferred over a passive warm-up (using external agents such as hot showers, saunas, or ultrasound). However, passive heating in the form of a hot shower may be indicated for people with severe arthritis before engaging in fitness activities. Consider the health and fitness levels of participants and the type of activity being performed when determining the length and intensity of the warm-up.

Generally, 10 to 15 minutes of low-intensity continuous movement and gentle range of motion activities provides a good warm-up for physically independent adults. Use activities that gradually elevate participants' heart rates to the lower limit of their predetermined exercise heart rate range (see p. 60). Use a longer warm-up (20 minutes) for a higher-intensity exercise program or for frail or unconditioned clients. Physically frail adults will benefit from continuous gentle movement of the arms and legs while seated. They may begin to perspire (a sign that internal temperature is rising) after very mild activity, so monitor responses carefully.

Never start an adult exercise class with stretching. Adults who have not been regularly physically active can have relatively stiff, inflexible tendons, ligaments, and muscles, and this increases their risk for muscle and tendon strain or tear. Save the stretching to increase range of motion until after the aerobics phase, when the body is warm.

Many different activities can be used to increase internal body temperature. Examples include walking (on land or in water), performing rhythmic movements while seated or standing, and using cardiovascular equipment such as stationary bikes or steppers. Whenever possible, incorporate large-muscle activities into the warm-up (performed at low intensity) that are the same or similar to those you plan to use later in class. For example, if you plan to push the arms overhead during aerobics, perform that exercise more slowly during the warm-up. Use the warm-up to introduce new movement sequences at a slow tempo and low intensity. This approach allows participants to learn and practice before performing the sequence at full tempo during the aerobic phase of class, reducing anxiety and helping them to be successful in movement. Refer to chapter 5 for specific warm-up sequences.

Cooling Down

The purpose of cooling down is to slowly decrease body temperature, heart rate, and respiration to preactivity levels. The cool-down is the warm-up in reverse and can include many of the same types of low-intensity, continuous movements. Continuous movement keeps the muscles contracting to help the body return venous blood from the extremities to the heart, resulting in decreased muscle soreness. A proper cool-down can also prevent exercise-related problems such as dizziness and possible cardiac irregularities that can occur in high-risk populations.

Stretching, relaxing, reinforcing social connections, and making a conscious transition to the rest of the day are important components of a cool-down. Plan enough time to ensure a proper cool-down, at least 5 minutes for the body to return to preactivity levels plus at least 10 minutes for

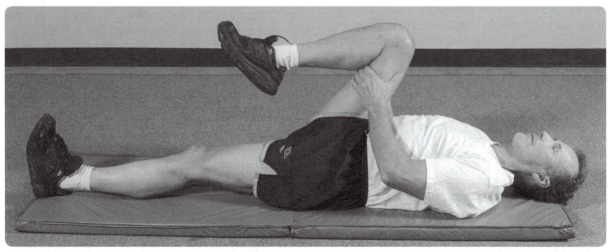

Encourage participants who can to stretch on a mat.

stretching and relaxation. The last stage of a cool-down should include exercises to increase range of motion. Stretches performed on a mat can benefit physically independent adults. For physically frail adults exercising in a chair, gradually reduce continuous movement patterns and systematically stretch all areas of the body, working from the head down. Incorporate relaxation strategies between stretches and at the end of class. Refer to chapter 5 for specific cool-down sequences.

Before all participants leave class, have them take one last pulse rate measurement or rate their perceived exertion level to ensure that recovery has occurred. Never allow a participant to leave class without a proper cool-down. Discourage participants from leaving class before completing a proper cool-down. Make it a standard policy that if people have to leave class early, they must complete their aerobic activities 10 minutes early and walk around the space (or reduce seated activity) until their heart rate, respiration, and body temperature have dropped. If someone leaves class unexpectedly, have an assistant or another class participant follow him to determine whether he is experiencing a health problem.

Aerobics

Considering the increased potential for cardiovascular dysfunction in the older adult population, you must use a variety of methods to ensure that participants are exercising at an appropriate aerobic level. Careful determination and monitoring of exercise intensity are the keys to safe aerobic activity. To monitor the aerobic phase, calculate each student's target heart rate zone and then check heart rates frequently. Train your students to evaluate their own ratings of perceived exertion and use this as a guideline in conjunction with the target heart rate guidelines. Get to know your participants so you will notice whether they look or act differently than normal, and be alert to any sudden change of behavior or appearance.

Determining Exercise Intensity

Participants need cardiovascular conditioning to maintain and improve function, but these activities must be performed at a safe level that allows gradual improvement. This can be achieved by determining safe, individual target heart rate zones and ratings of perceived exertion and having participants frequently check their heart rate responses to exercise. Teach students to recognize the signs of overexer-

tion, such as rapid breathing, loss of coordination, and flushed skin. Using this combination of methods helps participants discover exactly how intense their exercise should be.

Target Heart Rates Individual target heart rate zones can be determined using the Karvonen formula, which incorporates the participant's age and resting heart rate. However, it is unnecessary—and perhaps unwise—to push participants in a group class to reach 80% of their maximum heart rate, which is the standard high range of this formula. Research shows that even moderate- to low-intensity aerobic exercise provides a training benefit for most adults. A safe level for participants *without* heart disease is from 50% to 75% (see figure 4.2 for a modified Karvonen formula). Make certain that all participants know their target heart rates and understand what their 10-second counts should be. The accuracy of the Karvonen formula is challenged by the difficulty of knowing a participant's precise maximum heart rate and by the possibility for error in counting heart beats. For these reasons the rating of perceived exertion is a valuable tool to determine how hard participants believe they are working.

Participants with diagnosed heart disease should exercise at a heart rate recommended by their physicians and by their rating of perceived exertion. Some heart medications completely invalidate target heart rate calculations, so you must know which of your students take medication that necessitates use of the rating of perceived exertion instead of the Karvonen formula. Even for nonmedicated students, using the rating of perceived exertion coupled with the modified Karvonen formula to determine exercise intensity adds another measure of safety to the aerobic component of class.

Rating of Perceived Exertion Many medications artificially regulate the heart rate and thus invalidate target heart rate calculations. Therefore, students on these medications must not try to achieve a predetermined heart rate. Instead, they should rely on assessing their own rating of perceived exertion, which gauges how they feel during and after exercise.

To help exercisers determine rate of perceived exertion, ask them to answer the question "how hard am I working?" They should rate themselves using a 10-point scale with 1 being "very, very light" and 10 being "extremely hard." Exercisers should aim to achieve the moderate range (4 to 7) and be warned against working in the hardest range (8 to 10).

Resting heart rate (RHR)   To obtain an accurate RHR, count the pulse for 1 full minute after having been at complete rest for a minimum of 20 minutes.

Target heart rate (THR) zone   The average asymptomatic senior should be able to safely work between 50% and 75% of maximum heart rate (HR) during the aerobic phase.

10-second count   Count the pulse for 10 seconds to check heart rate during the aerobic phase.

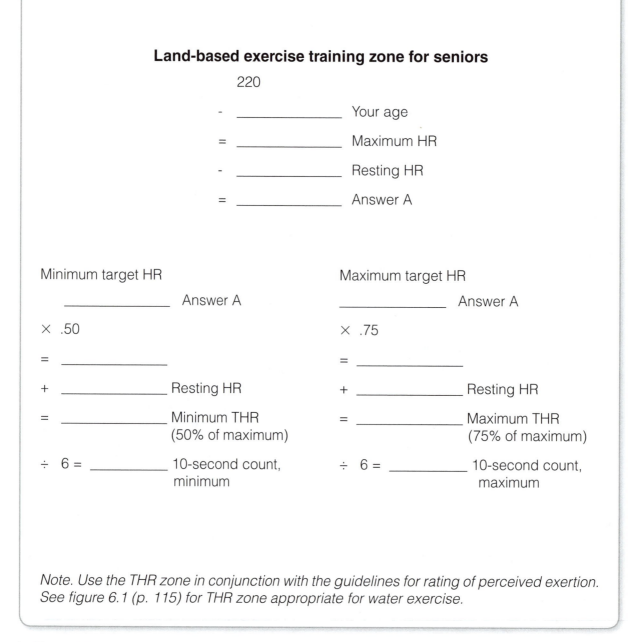

Land-based exercise training zone for seniors

220

- _____ Your age

= _____ Maximum HR

- _____ Resting HR

= _____ Answer A

Minimum target HR

_____ Answer A

× .50

= _____

+ _____ Resting HR

= _____ Minimum THR
(50% of maximum)

÷ 6 = _____ 10-second count,
minimum

Maximum target HR

_____ Answer A

× .75

= _____

+ _____ Resting HR

= _____ Maximum THR
(75% of maximum)

÷ 6 = _____ 10-second count,
maximum

Note. Use the THR zone in conjunction with the guidelines for rating of perceived exertion. See figure 6.1 (p. 115) for THR zone appropriate for water exercise.

▶ **Figure 4.2**   Modified Karvonen formula.

Another benefit of the rating of perceived exertion is its ability to provide important information about how participants are responding to exercise *that day*. The body's response to exercise is affected by many things, such as heat, cold, medications, stress, fatigue, or slight illness. Because of these and other factors, participants may actually be exercising below their target zones but feel like they are working hard. Giving the rating of perceived exertion equal importance to the calculated target heart rate zone will help ensure that participants are exercising at a safe level, that is, in line with their bodies' response to exercise that day.

Monitoring Exercise Intensity

Monitoring exercise intensity takes very little time but offers important feedback on how students are responding to exercise. Using a variety of techniques, both objective and subjective, will significantly increase the safety of your program.

To improve the reliability of heart rate checks, keep your method of checking the heart rate simple and consistent so that all class members can find and count their own pulse. Use the same cues each time you take an exercise pulse rate. Make the cues clear and direct: "Stop and find your pulse" (pause for 2-3 seconds); "ready, start" (count for 10 seconds); "stop." As soon as the 10-second count is completed, have participants march in place while each person tells you her or his 10-second count. Practice taking exercise pulse and recovery pulse rates with your students so they all feel comfortable with and confident about the procedure; with practice, each heart rate check will take only a few moments.

There is some disagreement about whether it is better to take the pulse at the carotid artery, which is on the neck, or at the brachial artery, on the wrist. A participant who has diminished feeling in the tips of the fingers may have difficulty finding and counting her pulse. Have participants try both the carotid and the brachial pulse points to determine which one works better for them.

The carotid pulse should be taken by placing the fingers of the right hand onto the right side of the neck close to the windpipe. Caution your students not to press too firmly on this spot—too much pressure could cause a person to become lightheaded. Also tell them to avoid reaching across the throat to the right side of the neck with the left hand or grasping at the windpipe area with the fingers on one side and the thumb on the other (and thus squeezing the windpipe). Both of these positions can restrict the flow of oxygen and cause lightheadedness.

The brachial pulse should be taken by placing the fingers (not the thumb) of the left hand onto the "thumb side" of the front of the right wrist (palm facing up). Firm pressure here will not cause a problem. Take the time to make sure that all students can find their pulses at one location or the other. If you rush through this procedure, it is likely that a higher percentage of participants will not take an accurate heart rate reading but will simply call out a number similar to the ones they hear around them. This can pose a danger because it sidesteps one of your primary methods of ensuring proper exercise intensity.

During the aerobic phase, have students practice determining their ratings of perceived exertion by asking each person to give you a number that indicates how hard each believes she is working according to the rating of perceived exertion (see page 59). Requiring each person to make this determination reemphasizes the importance of proper exercise intensity and the probability of differences between people in their response to exercise. It will also help participants who have difficulty finding and counting their pulse to find an exercise intensity that feels comfortable.

Frequent Heart Rate Checks During each class period, check heart rates before beginning (preexercise rate) and after the warm-up. This will tell participants how their bodies are responding to exercise that day. Then continue to monitor exercise intensity frequently by checking heart rates two or three times during the aerobic phase and asking each person for his 10-second count. Take note of participants who are on medications that artificially regulate heart rates, and ask all participants for their ratings of perceived exertion. This frequent checking can alert you immediately to potential problems.

At the end of the aerobic phase, check exercise heart rates again. Have everyone walk slowly for 1 minute and then take their recovery pulse for 10 seconds. Ask students how many beats they decreased in the 1-minute recovery period. If you have students whose pulse rates do not decrease after 1 minute, take their pulse again 1 minute later to determine whether it has decreased. Failure of the heart to recover noticeably after aerobic exercise can indicate a variety of problems. Monitor these participants throughout the rest of the class to determine whether their heart rates are responding. A participant whose heart rate goes overly high (heart rate 12-15 beats over that person's maximum target heart rate) and who does not recover promptly should consult his physician.

Before beginning the cool-down phase, again ask students, regardless of whether they are on heart rate medication, to indicate their ratings of perceived exertion. This will help your students become aware of how they feel when they are exercising within their own target heart rate zones.

Recording Exercise Intensity For easy referral, write each student's predetermined 10-second count or indicate her reliance on the rate of perceived exertion next to her name on a role sheet or chart. Keep a record of each student's exercise heart rate, recovery heart rate, and rating of perceived exertion for every exercise period during the first several weeks of class (see the sample chart in figure 4.3). Recording these figures will familiarize you with each person's response to exercise and alert you to any potential problems, such as excessively high exercise heart rates or failure of the heart to recover after 1 minute. This practice will also reinforce to your students the importance of monitoring exercise intensity with both the target heart rate and the rate of perceived exertion. After you become familiar with your class members and their responses to exercise, continue to ask each participant for these numbers even if you no longer take the time to record them.

Flexibility

Maintaining flexibility is critical to functional fitness, which is the level of fitness necessary for people to take care of their personal needs, maintain an independent lifestyle, and participate in activities they value. Therefore, aerobic classes should include a flexibility component after the initial cool-down (recovery phase). Design flexibility work that contributes to functional fitness by maintaining range of motion in all joints and promoting ease of movement. Your motto as an instructor should be "movement that matters." Think about the bending, stretching, and reaching that are necessary in any given day to maintain an independent lifestyle and prevent loss of function. These are movements that matter.

Give special attention to the areas that are typically troublesome for many adults—the upper back, neck and shoulders, low back, and hamstrings. The safest and most effective stretches are gentle and slow. Offer alternative exercises or modifications for stretches to take into account the high potential for muscle and joint dysfunction among older adult participants who have been sedentary. Protect the joints by avoiding stretches that place a joint in an awkward position, and instruct the class to keep the rest of the body as relaxed as possible while stretching a particular muscle group. See chapter 5 for land-based stretches and chapter 6 for water-based stretches.

Strength and Power

Strength is the amount of force a muscle can generate. Many adults who have been sedentary have a significantly diminished level of strength. Research indicates that a large percentage of adults 70 and older cannot lift and carry 10 pounds (Clark et al., 1998). Considering all of the things a person must lift and carry in the course of a day, you can see the large role strength plays in functional independence. Strength helps older people prevent muscle and joint injury, maintain balance, and prevent falls. This is of critical importance, because falls are a leading cause of accidental death among adults older than 65.

The latest research demonstrates that power (the ability to generate force quickly, or strength × speed) is even more critical to retaining function than strength alone. Consider how difficult it is to perform many functional tasks without the speed component. Try rising from a chair or climbing stairs very slowly, or imagine trying to catch your balance to prevent a fall without the necessary speed of contraction. Research shows that muscle power is lost at a faster rate than strength and is more closely associated with performance of the activities of daily living than is strength alone. Power training has proven more effective than strength training for improving physical function, so instructors must make a conscious effort to incorporate power training into programs. Muscle power can be increased with high-velocity training (Hazell et al., 2006; Miszko et al., 2003).

Resistance training (strength and power work) is crucial to retaining or regaining function and also builds confidence by offering rapid, readily noticeable results. Whenever possible, incorporate resistance work into classes by using stretchy bands, hand weights, body weight, or water resistance. Always warm up the class before strength training and involve major muscle groups of the lower and upper body. Train participants to protect their joints through proper alignment, smooth movements, and appropriate training intensity. When using resistance bands, ensure that participants are mindful of their wrist position to prevent hyperflexion of the wrist against resistance.

Power training requires high-velocity contractions (contracting the muscles as quickly as possible), so you must ensure that equipment and

Date																		
Name	EHR/R	RPE	EHR/R	RPE	EHR/R	RPE	EHR/R	RPE	EHR/R	RPE	EHR/R	RPE	EHR/R	RPE	EHR/R	RPE	EHR/R	RPE

EHR = exercise heart rate; R = recovery heart rate; RPE = rating of perceived exertion.

▲ **Figure 4.3** Record-keeping chart.

From K. Van Norman, 2010, *Exercise and wellness for older adults*, 2nd ed. (Champaign, IL: Human Kinetics).

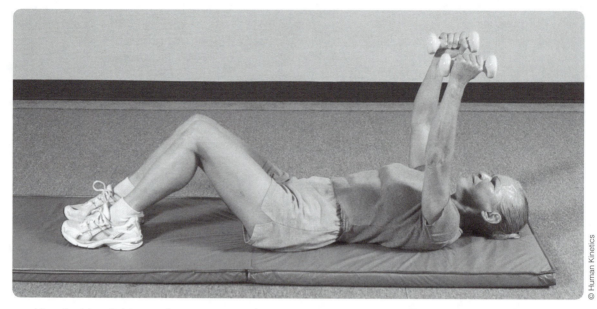

Handheld weights can improve strength.

movement strategies safely allow speed of movement. For example, an exercise machine with an iron weight stack poses a problem for training power because the protocol of a 2- or 3-second lift (to control momentum of the weight stack) makes it virtually impossible to train for power. Refer to chapter 5 for specific strength- and power-training protocols and exercises and a discussion of the types of equipment conducive to training power.

Coordination and Balance

Coordination and balance are vital in maintaining physical function. Both play a large role in the prevention of falls and can deteriorate rapidly if not practiced. Coordination can be easily addressed in classes through unison and opposition work,

sequencing of movements, and an endless variety of arm and leg combinations. Balance activities can easily be done in the water (especially good for those with compromised balance), such as rising onto toes, transferring weight to one foot while lifting the other off the pool bottom, or rocking forward onto the toes and back onto the heels. In land-based exercise, balance work can be done standing in circles, holding hands for support, or standing next to a wall or chair (see chapters 5 and 6).

Practicing balance and coordination will increase your participants' confidence in movement. Participants' self-esteem will be enhanced as balance and coordination activities become progressively easier to perform. An excellent resource for balance training is *Fall Proof: A Comprehensive Balance and Mobility Training Program* (Rose, 2003).

WELLNESS WRAP-UP

A quality program requires a well-trained instructor, good class organization and management, and attention to safety. It also requires a well-rounded program that identifies levels of function and needs, offers safe exercises and movement sequences, and addresses psychosocial aspects of well-being. Consciously designing class elements to support social and emotional elements of well-being embraces the concept and intent of whole-person wellness. Well-designed programs can improve participants' confidence in their abilities and self-esteem and offer important social connections. An exercise class must include a warm-up and a cool-down and as many of the other components of fitness as possible, including carefully monitored aerobic training and activities to promote strength and power, flexibility, coordination, and balance.

Land-Based Programming

A variety of land-based classes can meet the needs of participants across the range of functional abilities. This chapter offers specific techniques for warming up and cooling down, chair and chair-assisted exercise, low-impact aerobics, and strength and power training. The exercises are described and illustrated with photographs, and sample class outlines demonstrate how to put the exercises together into a 1-hour class. In addition, this chapter describes the concept of whole-person wellness stations, which are designed to provide clients with self-directed opportunities to improve well-being in multiple dimensions of health. The chapter provides ideas for making and using inexpensive exercise props.

Regardless of participants' level of functional ability, class should begin the moment clients enter the room. Many clients will come early to walk around the space or visit with other participants and the instructor. This time can serve as a "pre-warm-up" in multiple dimensions; it's a great time to get participants fully involved in the class, engaging them physically but also connecting them socially and emotionally to other participants and the instructor. Making this time before class a priority contributes significantly to the whole-person wellness approach of your program. Greet and welcome everyone to class. Introduce new participants to the group and to individuals, and ask a long-time member to act as a new participant's "sponsor." This will help newcomers feel like a part of the group even before the class begins.

CHAIR EXERCISE

Chair exercise can vary in intensity from vigorous chair aerobics designed to provide aerobic benefits for healthy adults to movement that concentrates on maintaining a basic level of function for frail participants. This chapter addresses the low to middle levels of intensity. Techniques described consist of chair and chair-assisted exercise designed to improve range of motion, strength, coordination, and balance. Strategies are also provided that promote socialization and fun and allow participants to gain confidence in physical activity.

The target population for low- to mid-level chair exercise includes physically dependent, frail, or chair-bound adults; those with joint problems or significant balance deficits; and those with cardiovascular or respiratory diseases that preclude participation in aerobic activity. Primarily healthy but very sedentary or overweight adults can ben-efit from chair exercise that helps them regain confidence in their ability to be physically active. Participants can remain seated during any of the chair-assisted activities. An excellent resource for chair exercise is Mary Ann Wilson, RN, of the *Sit and Be Fit* program aired on public television. She has a large variety of programs for multiple levels of ability and specialized programs for adults with specific health conditions. Visit her site at www.sitandbefit.org.

Cautions

Adults who are physically dependent or frail are at high risk for osteoporosis. Therefore, certain movements should be avoided or used sparingly in chair exercise. Avoid all jerky, ballistic movements and rapid twisting or turning of any body part. Avoid excessive compression of the abdominal area, especially for those participants who show evidence of spinal compression (forward curvature of the spine). Bending all the way over at the waist can put stress on internal organs that may already be crowded. Similarly, standing on one leg exerts a great deal of pressure on the hip joint, which could also be dramatically weakened by osteoporosis. To protect the hip joint, avoid having participants stand on one leg for more than 8 counts, and avoid any twisting motion of the hip while participants are standing on one leg. People who are in the later stages of osteoporosis should avoid exercising while standing on one leg.

Movement That Matters

Focus on movement that matters by identifying movements that participants need to perform easily to take care of their personal needs, known as activities of daily living or ADLs, including self-feeding, toileting, dressing, transferring, and walking. Include exercises that improve strength in the quadriceps muscles, which allow people to rise from and lower onto chairs, get into and out of bed, and use the toilet without assistance. To remain independent, people must be able to lift and carry things of various sizes and weights. Exercising with resistance bands or 1- to 5-pound weights can improve upper-body strength; heavier weights can be used for the legs. Look for variable-resistance weights that allow participants to gradually increase resistance as they get stronger. If you have access to strength training machines, refer to subsequent sections in this chapter for exercises and strategies to move your participants from training with handheld weights to machine training.

Include upper-body mobility exercises to help participants maintain the ability to comb their hair, dress themselves, and take care of other personal needs. Ask participants which everyday activities they would like to be able to perform more easily, and then build a program that addresses these tasks.

Repeat each exercise 4 to 12 times, depending on participants' level of ability, and add resistance only once they are successful in movement. See table 4.1 (p. 54) for a list of levels of function, needs, and recommended activities.

▶ Specific Chair Exercises

To create a well-balanced exercise series, start from the top of the head and work down through the body, concentrating on moving each joint through its appropriate range of motion. Perform all exercises gently, completing each full range of motion slowly and smoothly. Routinely remind participants to breathe normally throughout all of the exercises. Count slowly for all exercises and provide extra reminders to breathe normally while holding a stretched position. Include a short section of continuous movements like knee lifts, arm swings, and small kicks done to upbeat music to improve endurance. The duration will depend on your group, but most people should be able to perform 5 minutes of endurance exercise. Encourage participants to work at their own pace, and gradually increase this segment of class as appropriate.

In the following exercises, the neutral position is sitting up straight in the chair with the shoulders directly over the hips (the spine is not relaxed into the back of the chair), facing forward, shoulders square to front, arms hanging relaxed at the sides, head and neck centered, feet flat on the floor. All exercises begin in the neutral position unless otherwise specified.

Neck Exercises

CAUTION: **Do not ask exercisers to lift the chin past neutral or drop the head back. This can cause cervical compression and dizziness. Avoid all rapid or jerky movements with the neck.**

- **Ear to Shoulder:** Exercisers gently lower right ear toward right shoulder, return to neutral; lower left ear toward left shoulder, return to neutral, lower chin toward the chest, and return to neutral. Hold each position for 8 to 12 counts. Remind exercisers to keep shoulders down in a relaxed position and breathe normally throughout the exercise.

- **Neck Rotation:** Participants look over right shoulder, return to neutral, look over the left shoulder, return to neutral, pull the chin back (keeping head level), and return to neutral. Perform each movement to a slow 8 counts.

- ▶ **Neck Stretch:** With the palm of the right hand on the right side of head, exercisers use the neck muscles to push against the hand with the head for 4 to 8 counts and then release the hand and relax the neck to neutral (figure 5.1). Gently lower the left ear to the left shoulder and hold for 8 counts; return to neutral. Repeat the exercise with the left palm on the left side of the head.

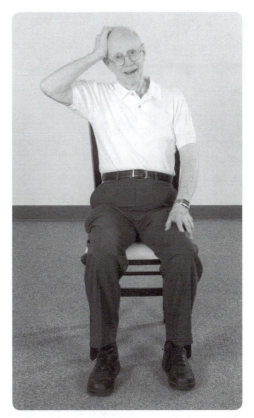

▶ **Figure 5.1** Neck stretch.

- **Nose Circle:** Exercisers slowly draw small circles in the air with their noses 3 or 4 times clockwise and then 3 or 4 times counterclockwise (8 counts for each circle).

Shoulder and Upper-Back Exercises

CAUTION: Exercisers must avoid dropping the arms forcefully from a position above the head or out to the sides. After the shoulders are lifted, the return to neutral should be slow and controlled.

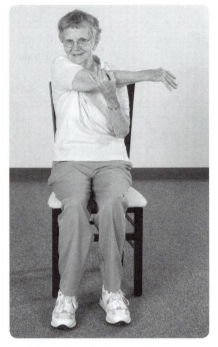

▶ **Figure 5.2** Cross arm.

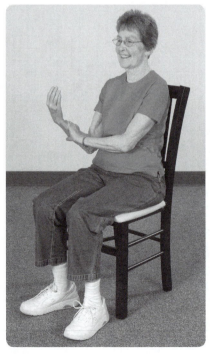

▶ **Figure 5.3** Biceps curl.

- **Shoulder Shrugs:** Exercisers lift both shoulders to ears, return to neutral; press shoulders down, and return to neutral, using 4 counts for each movement.
- **Shoulder Lifts:** Participants lift right shoulders up, left shoulders up; right shoulders down, left shoulders down (1 count each). Then move both shoulders up and both shoulders down (2 counts each).
- **Shoulder Circles:** Exercisers move one shoulder (or both) in circular motion, forward or backward, 4 to 8 counts for each circle.
- **Blade Squeeze:** Exercisers round shoulders forward (4 counts), return to neutral (4 counts), pull shoulders backward so shoulder blades squeeze together in back (hold for 8 counts), and then return to neutral (4 counts).
- **Squeeze and Stretch:** With hands on shoulders, elbows out, participants touch elbows together in front (4 counts) and return to neutral (4 counts). Then they press elbows toward the back so that the shoulder blades are squeezed together (8 counts) and return to neutral (4 counts).
- **Arm Reaches:** Using one or both arms in any combination and the hands returning to touch the shoulder between each reach, exercisers reach out to sides, hands to shoulders; reach overhead, hands to shoulders; reach forward, hands to shoulders; reach down, hands to shoulders.
- ◀ **Cross Arm:** Exercisers reach right arm across the front of the chest to the left and then hold the right forearm with the left hand and gently stretch (not jerk or tug) the right shoulder for 8 to 12 counts (figure 5.2). Instruct participants to keep their shoulder blades squeezed together in back during the stretch. Then participants release the right arm, sweep it around to the front of the body, and return it to neutral (4 counts). Repeat the stretch with left arm crossing the chest to the right.

Elbow, Wrist, and Hand Exercises

◀ **Biceps Curl:** With hands on thighs, palms facing up, exercisers flex their elbows and touch their hands to their shoulders (figure 5.3), alternating right and left hands or using both at the same time. To increase biceps strength, exercisers place the left hand on the right forearm and push down, resisting the right biceps curl, and repeat with the left arm. A stretchy band or light weight can be used for resistance. Avoid shoulder impingement by keeping the elbows in front of the body in any upper-body strength moves that involve the shoulder joint.

■ **Curl and Touch:** With hands on thighs, palms facing up, exercisers flex the right elbow, touch the right hand to the right shoulder, reach the right arm overhead and touch the right hand to the left shoulder, reach the right arm overhead again and touch the right hand to the right shoulder, and return hand to thigh, palm facing up. Repeat using left hand (1 count for each movement). Finally, repeat the movement using both right and left hands at the same time.

■ **Prayer Hands:** Exercisers press palms together in praying position (4 counts), slowly lift the elbows out to the sides until the wrists flex to approximately 90 degrees (4 counts), hold for 4 counts, and then bring elbows down in 4 counts.

■ **Wrist Circles:** Exercisers rotate wrist in circles, with open hands and then with hands closed into fists.

■ **Finger Fan:** Exercisers close the hands to fists, open and spread the fingers apart, close extended fingers together like closing a fan, open and spread fingers apart, close fingers, and then close the hands to fists (2-4 counts for each movement).

■ **Finger Drawing:** Exercisers draw circles in the air with one finger at a time on both hands (i.e., both thumbs and then index, middle, ring, and pinky fingers). Alternate directions and use the full range of motion. For variety, have exercisers write in the air with each finger.

■ **Finger Pinch:** Exercisers pinch the index finger and thumb together to form a circle; repeat with each finger (1 count for each). Then they close their hands into fists (2 counts), and open and spread their fingers wide (2 counts). A gel ball or sponge can be pinched between the index finger and thumb to add resistance.

Torso Exercises

Participants should perform all torso exercises while sitting up straight in the neutral position without dipping the shoulders to the right or left.

■ **Torso Isolations:** Exercisers shift the torso to the right side, return to neutral, shift to the left side, return to neutral (2 counts each); push torso to the front, return to neutral, pull to the back, return to neutral (2 counts each); then make a full circle right (8 counts) and a full circle left (8 counts).

▶ **Contraction:** Exercisers round the back (but not by sinking down or slumping in their chairs), press grasped hands forward for 8 counts (figure 5.4), and then slowly straighten the back while opening the arms out to sides and then lowering them to the neutral position over 8 counts.

■ **Rotation:** Exercises gently turn to the right and, twisting at the waist, look over the right shoulder (turn 4 counts, hold 8 counts); they return to neutral (4 counts) and repeat the movement to the left.

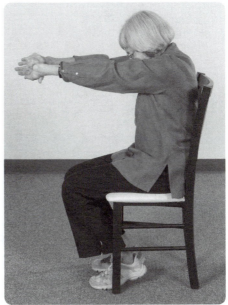

▶ **Figure 5.4** Contraction.

CAUTION: Be sure participants' feet are flat on the floor at least shoulder-width apart while doing this exercise. This will prevent them from reaching too far and losing balance. Use the image of pulling on a rope to draw something toward themselves.

■ **Reach and Pull:** With the right arm, exercisers reach as far across to the left side of the body as possible. They tighten the arm muscles as if grasping something and pulling it toward themselves while returning the arm to neutral using 4 counts; using the left arm, exercisers reach to the left and grasp and pull while returning to neutral. They repeat the movement with the left arm reaching across the right side of the body and pulling back to neutral and then the right arm reaching to the right and pulling back to neutral, again for 4 counts each.

■ **Deep Breaths:** Exercisers take a deep breath, fully expanding the abdomen, and then blow the air out slowly and evenly; repeat. Emphasize filling the lungs to their fullest capacity each time and then expelling air completely.

Hip Exercises

These exercises should be done in the neutral position, except the participants should relax their spines against the back of the chair to allow for more freedom of movement in the hip socket.

▼ **Leg Cross:** Exercisers lift the right leg (knee bent) straight up (counts 1, 2), cross it over the left knee (3, 4), bring the right leg back to center (5, 6), and then return to neutral position (7, 8); repeat with the left leg crossing right (figure 5.5). Participants who have had a recent hip replacement should avoid this exercise.

■ **Leg Open Side:** Exercisers lift the right leg (knee bent) straight up (counts 1, 2), open to the right side (3, 4), close to center (5, 6), and return to neutral (7, 8); repeat with the left leg opening to the left side.

▼ **Hip Rotation:** Participants extend the right leg to the front with the foot flexed, rotate the leg out from the hip, return to center, rotate in, and return to center (figure 5.6). (This rotation will be small, occurring at the hip, not the knee or ankle.) Repeat 4 times before returning leg to neutral. Then repeat the whole series with the left leg.

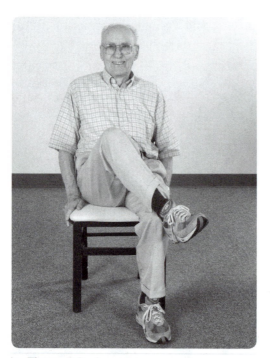

▶ **Figure 5.5** Leg cross.

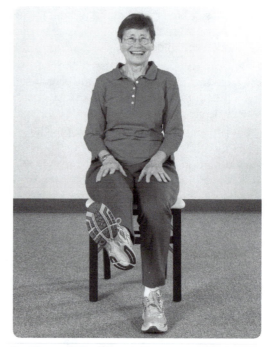

▶ **Figure 5.6** Hip rotation.

CAUTION: Instruct participants to keep the back straight while performing the following knee lifts and to twist in a slow, controlled manner.

■ **Knee Lifts:** Exercisers do alternating knee lifts to the front, touching right hand to right knee and left hand to left knee, or do cross-knee lifts, touching the left elbow to the right knee and the right elbow to the left knee, 1 count for each movement. Return to neutral after each knee lift.

■ **Double Knee Lifts:** Exercisers lift the right knee to the front and then return to neutral. Lift right knee to the front again and return to neutral. Repeat, lifting the left knee 2 times.

▶ **Hip Stretch:** Exercisers carefully place the right ankle on the left knee, gently press down on the inside of the right knee to stretch the right hip (figure 5.7) (the right leg will be rotated to the right at the hip with the knee pointing to the side), hold the stretch for 8 counts, and then return to neutral. Repeat the movement on the left side with the left ankle resting on the right knee.

CAUTION: This exercise should not be done by anyone who feels tension or pain in the knee while in the stretched position or by those with a recent hip replacement.

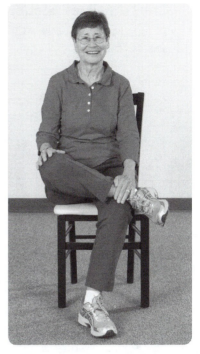

▶ **Figure 5.7** Hip stretch.

Knee, Ankle, and Feet Exercises

CAUTION: Whenever the legs are extended to the front, be sure that participants keep their abdominal muscles engaged and backs straight with no hyperextension of the low back.

■ **Knee Extensions:** Using 2 counts for each movement, participants extend the right leg to the front and then flex the knee back to neutral. Repeat 4 to 8 times right and then repeat with the left leg. To promote quadriceps strength, use ankle weights or have exercisers cross the left ankle over the right so that when the right leg is extending to the front, it is also lifting the weight of the left leg; repeat with the other leg.

■ **Extend and Point:** Exercisers extend the right leg to the front (counts 1, 2), point the toe (3, 4), flex the foot (5, 6), and point (7, 8); flex (1, 2), point (3, 4), flex (5, 6), and return to neutral (7, 8). Repeat with the left leg.

■ **Extend and Circle:** Participants extend the right leg to the front, perform right ankle circles in each direction using the full range of motion (allow 8 counts for each circle), and return to neutral; repeat with the left leg. To promote quadriceps strength, increase the time that the leg remains extended to the front (e.g., do points, flexes, and ankle circles; turn foot in and then turn it out) before returning to neutral.

■ **Ankle Rocks:** Exercisers rise up onto their toes and then press their heels down to a flat foot; they rock back onto both heels, pulling their toes off the floor, and then press down to a flat foot. Use 2 counts for each movement.

■ **Toe Curls:** Keeping the sole of their foot on the floor, exercisers do toe curls (i.e., grip the floor with the toes), return to neutral, pull toes up and back (off the floor), and then return to neutral. Allow 2 counts for each movement.

■ **Toe Taps:** Keeping the heels on the floor, exercisers do alternating toe taps while flexing the ankle as far as possible each time (they will feel the muscles in the front of the shin), 1 count for each tap. Instead of alternating, participants may do 8 to 10 toe taps with the right foot before changing to the left.

Chair-Assisted Standing Exercises

There are three main positions for chair-assisted exercises: standing directly behind the chair with both hands on the chair back (neutral) (figure 5.8a), standing to the right of the chair with the left hand on the chair back (right-side neutral) (figure 5.8b), and standing to the left side of the chair with the right hand on the chair back (left-side neutral) (figure 5.8c). The hands should only rest lightly on the chair. Caution your participants not to lean on the chair or rely solely on it for balance.

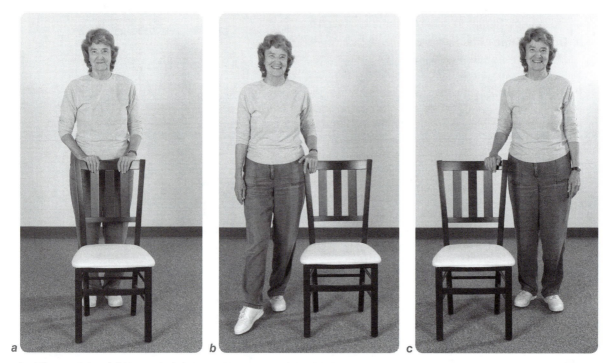

a   b   c

▶ **Figure 5.8** *(a)* Neutral; *(b)* right-side neutral; *(c)* left-side neutral.

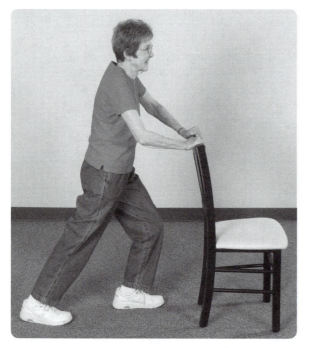

▶ **Figure 5.9** Achilles stretch.

- **Rise-Up:** Standing in neutral position, exercisers rise up onto their toes (counts 1, 2), hold (3, 4, 5, 6), and then bring their heels down (7, 8).

- **Knee Bends:** Standing in neutral position and keeping both feet flat on the floor, exercisers bend both knees (counts 1, 2), hold (3, 4, 5, 6), and then straighten legs (7, 8). Participants should keep the back straight throughout the exercise and bend the knees directly over the toes.

- Use rise-ups and knee bends in a variety of sequences; for example, rise up (counts 1, 2), hold (3, 4, 5, 6), bring heels down (7, 8), bend knees (counts 1, 2), hold (3, 4, 5, 6), and straighten legs (7, 8).

- ◀ **Achilles Stretch:** In the lunge position with the left leg forward, exercisers press the right heel to the floor (figure 5.9), hold for 8 to 12 counts, and return to neutral. Repeat on the opposite side in the lunge position with the right leg forward. Keep the hips square to the front, front knee bent, and back leg straight.

- **Hamstring Contraction:** Standing in neutral position, exercisers flex the knee and lift the right heel toward the right buttock (counts 1, 2), hold (3, 4, 5, 6), return to neutral (7, 8), and repeat, lifting the left heel toward the left buttock. This movement can be done as a double heel lift: Exercisers flex and lift the right heel 2 times, return to neutral position, flex and lift the left knee 2 times, and then return to neutral position. Instruct exercisers to contract their muscles to lift the heel rather than fling the heel toward the buttock. Ankle weights can be added for resistance.

▶ **Press-Backs:** Beginning in neutral position, exercisers lift the right heel until the knee is flexed to 90 degrees (figure 5.10) (counts 1, 2), press the right leg back 2 times, keeping the knee flexed and the back straight (3, 4 and 5, 6), and then return to neutral (7, 8). Repeat with the left leg.

- **Touch-Outs:** Beginning in right-side neutral position, exercisers reach out with the right toe to touch front (counts 1, 2), touch side (3, 4), touch back (5, 6), and return to neutral position (7, 8). Then they bend their knees, keeping heels on the floor (1, 2), straighten the legs (3, 4), bend knees (5, 6), and straighten legs (7, 8). Repeat exercise on right except touch toe back, toe side, toe front, and return to neutral position; then instead of bending knees on counts 1 to 2, rise onto the toes, lower heels (3, 4), rise onto toes (5, 6), and lower heels (7, 8). Repeat the entire sequence using the left leg beginning in left-side neutral position.

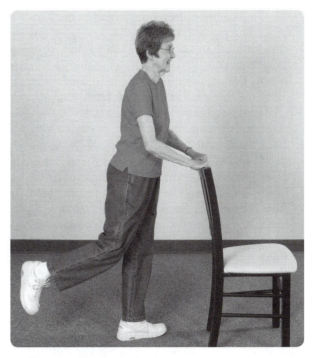

▶ **Figure 5.10** Press-backs.

Using Props and Equipment With Chair Exercise

Props add interest, variety, and fun to chair exercise. Many low-cost items can be both beneficial and fun to use. You can make 1- to 3-pound hand weights from PVC pipe and lead shot from a hardware store. You can also make small ankle weights from sturdy material filled with shot that can wrap around the ankle and also fit into the hands. Resistance bands are widely available from fitness supply catalogs and can be used in a variety of ways. Yarn balls and homemade rackets made from old nylon stockings stretched over metal coat hangers can be used for game activities. Look through books on elementary-school physical education programming for more ideas on making low-cost equipment. Many common items can be used in your exercise classes—just use your imagination.

Koosh Balls and Sponges

Koosh balls, found in many toy stores and large discount stores, are wonderful props for chair exercise. They are light and easy to handle, have an interesting feel, and can be easily squeezed in one hand. Use them to exercise the hand and fingers. Try a variety of sequences, such as squeeze 8 times right hand, 8 times left hand, 4 times right, 4 times left, 2 times right, 2 times left, 1 time right, 1 time left.

Koosh balls are easy to toss up in the air and catch, because they will not bounce off a person's hands like a tennis or foam ball. To improve coordination, have participants toss the ball up and clap one or two times before catching it again. Or use the balls in partner work where participants sit across from each other and toss one or two balls back and forth.

Koosh balls rolled up and down the legs and arms and between the hands provide tactile stimulation and improve circulation. You can also use these balls to exercise the feet. Rolling a ball back and forth with the bare sole of the foot provides a wonderful foot massage. Participants can also attempt to pick the ball up from the floor with their toes.

Sponges of various sizes and shapes can be squeezed, tossed, and gripped with the toes. Small sponges can be squeezed or wrung in the hands or rolled and squeezed with the feet and toes. Sponges can be used in toss-and-catch games, although they bounce off the hands easily. Large sponges (for washing automobiles) can be placed under the arms and squeezed to work the shoulder and upper-arm muscles, between the knees to work the inner thigh muscles, or behind the low back to work the abdominal muscles (flatten the sponge against the back of the chair by contracting the abdominals). Have participants place a large sponge under the ball of the foot, flatten the sponge against the floor, and then release it by flexing the ankles. Having a prop makes it much easier for participants to understand what it means to flex the ankle (i.e., when they pull their toes up off of the sponge, they are flexing their ankles).

Wooden Dowels and Scarves

Wooden dowels can be used in stretching and strength-promoting exercises. Have participants hold the dowel at shoulder level (in front of the body with hands approximately 8-10 inches [20-25 centimeters] apart, palms facing out), push it over the head (counts 1 and 2), hold (3, 4), pull the dowel down to chest level (5, 6), and hold (7, 8); Repeat 2 counts of 8. Participants can also exercise their wrists by turning the dowel forward or backward in their hands, first with palms facing down and then with palms facing up.

Dowels can be used for standing exercises. Exercisers can place one end onto the floor and walk or even do a step–kick sequence around the dowel to upbeat music. Use your imagination to come up with simple, safe routines appropriate for your group.

Scarves can be used to improve hand agility. Have each participant hold a relatively long scarf by the corner with the right hand, and then, using the fingers of the right hand only, wad the scarf up into a ball. Repeat with the left hand. Scarves can be tossed in the air and caught, and multiple scarves can be used for a slow version of juggling.

An alternative is to use the right hand to roll up a sheet of newspaper into a ball (just like with the scarf). Next have participants transfer the ball to their left hands and then, using only the left hand, uncrumple the newspaper ball. Participants then switch sides, crumpling the paper with the left hand and uncrumpling with the right hand.

Resistance Bands, Ankle Weights, and Handheld Weights

Resistance bands are made of a stretchy material and come in a variety of strengths, from light resistance to heavy resistance. Light- to medium-resistance bands usually are most appropriate for chair exercise. Some bands are made of a flat material, some are made of tubing, and some have handles to grip. Resistance bands can be ordered from most fitness supply catalogs either precut or in bulk rolls that allow you to measure and cut the band to the size you need.

Ankle weights are available in a wide range of resistance and can be used with most of the leg exercises described in this section. Start with weights ranging from 3 to 8 pounds or ankle weights that allow you to increase the resistance by adding weight as participants become stronger. Add weight to an exercise only if the participants are easily performing it without weight. Instruct participants to keep the body in alignment while performing the exercises and only lift the weight through the pain-free range of motion. Do not add weight to an exercise if it would require an awkward body position or to exercises where the legs are swinging (e.g., rhythmic coordination exercises).

Handheld weights are available in a wide range of resistance. Again, most of the exercises described in this section can be performed with weights, but only add weights if the participants are easily able to perform the exercise without weights. Ensure proper body alignment and instruct participants to perform only through the pain-free range of motion; do not add weight to exercises where the arms are swinging (e.g., rhythmic coordination exercises).

Resistance Band Exercises

Resistance bands can be used to develop both upper- and lower-body strength. When working on upper-body strength, be sure your participant keeps her elbow next to or in front of, rather than behind, her body. To avoid painful impingement of the shoulder joint (pinching the ligaments in the joint), keep the elbow in front of the body while performing strength moves involving the shoulder joint. A strip of resistance band approximately 3 feet (about 1 meter) long works well for the following exercises. Frequently remind exercisers to hold the band properly by keeping the wrist locked straight rather than flexed either forward or backward.

▶ **Biceps Curl:** Exercisers place the right foot on one end of the band and grip the other end with the right hand, keeping the wrist locked straight (avoid hyperextending the wrist), and then flex the elbow to bring the right hand to the right shoulder (biceps curl) (figure 5.11). The number of repetitions will depend on the strength of the participants and the resistance of the band (4-10 times is a good range). Repeat for the left arm.

■ **Chest Press:** Have participants place the band behind the back and grasp one end of the band with the right hand and the other end with the left hand. With elbows touching their sides, they slowly push their arms out to the front to extend the elbows and then slowly flex their elbows to bring them back to the starting position.

▼ **Triceps Press:** Participants grasp one end of the band with the right hand against the chest. They grasp the other end of the band with the left hand (6-8 inches [15-20 centimeters] from the right hand). Keeping the left elbow just below shoulder level and the forearm parallel to the floor, exercisers press the left hand forward, extending the elbow (figure 5.12). Then they slowly return to the starting position. Repeat 4 to 10 times, and then repeat with the left arm.

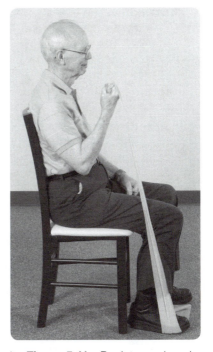

▶ **Figure 5.11** Resistance band biceps curl.

▼ **Upper-Back Row:** Participants place one end of the band under one foot grip the other end, and, with their elbows extended straight down and palms facing back, flex the elbows and pull toward the back (avoid pulling elbows behind the back) (figure 5.13), and then lower slowly to a straight arm. This can also be done with both arms at once by placing the middle of the band under both feet. Participants should do 4 to 8 repetitions.

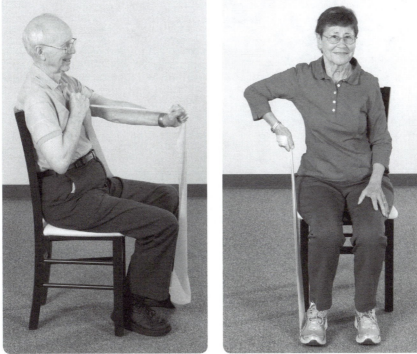

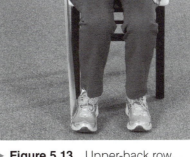

▶ **Figure 5.12** Triceps press.

▶ **Figure 5.13** Upper-back row.

▼ **Brake Push:** Participants place the left foot in the middle of the band and grasp one end with the right hand and one end with the left hand. They bring the left knee up toward the chest and pull their elbows to the sides (figure 5.14). Keeping elbows at the sides, participants push down with the left foot, extend the left knee (similar to a driver stepping on the brake pedal), and then slowly flex the knee again to return to the starting position. The number of repetitions (4-12) will depend on a participant's quadriceps and arm strength. Repeat the entire sequence with the right leg.

▼ **Knee Extension:** The exerciser ties the ends of the band into a bow (forming a circle or loop), places the loop around the right ankle, and then puts the left foot into the loop in front of the right foot (for best results, the right foot should be slightly back under the chair) (figure 5.15). Participants should perform 4 to 12 left knee extensions while keeping the right leg stationary (as an anchor point). Repeat the exercise with the left leg as the anchor point and the right leg performing the knee extensions.

CAUTION: Instruct participants *not* to stand up with the feet inside the band.

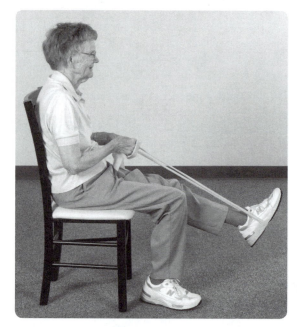

▶ **Figure 5.14**   Brake push.

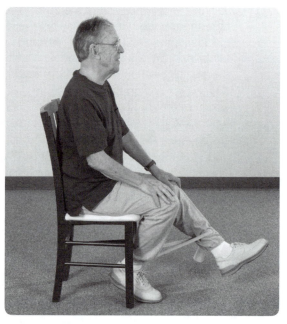

▶ **Figure 5.15**   Knee extension.

Coordination and Rhythmic Activities

You can use a variety of arm movements with simple leg movements to promote coordination. For example, using the same-side (i.e., unison) arm and leg, exercisers touch the right foot to the front while pushing or swinging the right arm forward and then return to neutral (allow 1 count for each move) (figure 5.16*a*). Repeat using the left foot and arm. Then touch the right foot to the right side while pushing or swinging both arms to the right side and return to neutral (1 count each); repeat using the left foot and both arms. For variation, use opposition (figure 5.16*b*): Exercisers move the right foot forward while the left arm pushes or swings forward and then return both to neutral position (1 count each); then they move the left foot forward while the right arm pushes or swings forward and return to neutral (1 count each). Next, participants move the right foot to the right side while both arms swing to the left, return to neutral, then move the left foot to the left side while both arms swing to the right, and return to neutral (1 count each).

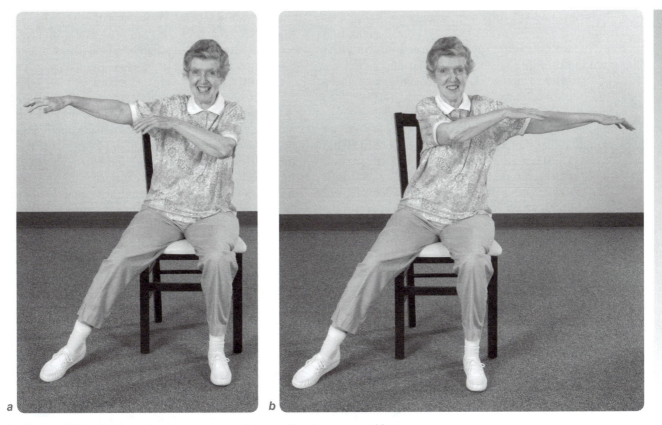

▶ **Figure 5.16** *(a)* Coordination—unison; *(b)* coordination—opposition.

Using unison and opposition movements, you can create an endless variety of arm and leg exercises that require both concentration and coordination to perform. Create short routines that your participants can learn and practice, and then set the routines to music everyone likes. Being able to complete a challenging routine gives students a boost in self-esteem, and it's fun! Visit www.kayvannorman .com for a video demonstrating a chair exercise class.

CAUTION: Do not add weight to swinging arms and legs.

Many rhythmic activities can be modified for chair exercise. You can use folk and square dance patterns by marching in place and using knee lifts instead of the normal traveling steps. For coordination activities, you can develop movements to be performed in 8-count, 4-count, and 2-count sets. For example, 8 toe touches forward, 8 heel presses forward, 8 touches to alternating sides, 8 kicks forward, and 8 knee lifts; then repeat the sequence using 4 counts of each, 2 counts of each, and 1 count of each.

Fun and Socialization

It is fun to use imagery during class. To "go for a walk in the forest," the class mimics movements such as walking up a steep incline, running from a bear, climbing a tree, or picking up pine cones. You can either make up the story yourself or ask each participant to contribute one movement for the story. This provides a great opportunity for interaction and engages participants physically, socially, and cognitively. You can also act out a familiar rhyme, like "The Noble Duke of York." to promote quadriceps strength for maintaining the ability to easily rise from and sit down on chairs. For example, seated in neutral position begin marching in place and reciting, "The noble Duke of York, he had 10,000 men, he marched them *up* the hill and marched them *down* again. When they were *up* they were up, and when they were *down* they were down, and when they were only *halfway up*, they were neither *up* nor *down*." Each time they say "up," participants stand up, and each time they say "down," they sit back down. At the phrase "when they were only halfway up," participants stand up into a crouched position, knees slightly bent, straightening the knees fully only at the next "up." Use your imagination to incorporate other rhymes with action words that could promote movement that matters.

Set aside time in class for socialization. Periodically have participants face each other and do partner work. This is especially easy with resistance bands. For example, have partners sit close together facing each other, one holding the ends of the band and the other holding the middle. Have the partner holding the ends do 8 to 10 upper-back rows (pulling elbows back) as the other partner holds the band steady. Then have the partner holding the middle do the rows while the person holding the ends holds the band steady. You can also do children's hand games like clapping and reaching across to partners in various rhythms. Take time at the end of class to encourage everyone to share news about what's happening with their family, their friends, or themselves. This is an excellent time to share special thoughts for the day, short poems, or inspirational writings, which can be found in small booklets in many stores. When this becomes a regular part of class, many participants will bring things they have heard or read to share with their classmates.

STANDING EXERCISE

Many chair-exercise participants will be able to progress to standing exercises. If participants are easily able to perform the exercises described in the previous section while standing behind or beside the chair, they may also be successful in programs incorporating walking, station work, wall work, and standing rhythmic exercises.

Follow the precautions for those with osteoporosis outlined in the chair-exercise portion of this chapter. Avoid quick changes of direction or rapid, jerky movements while walking or performing rhythmic exercises. Avoid exercises that require people to stand on one leg for more than 8 counts at a time and movements that involve twisting while standing on one leg.

Walking Courses

Walking is an excellent exercise and one of the most popular. To add interest and fun to your class, set up a walking course inside or outside of the building. Mark distances throughout the course so participants can keep track of their efforts both in class and on their own time. Remind walkers to practice "walking proud" by using their best posture and keeping eyes forward (rather than looking down). Participants who are unsteady in their gait can use handrails, if available, in hallways while still concentrating on good balance and keeping their eyes forward.

Record the distance everyone walks and give participants credit for this distance on a charted course. For example, the class may decide that they want to "walk across America." Each unit of distance participants walk (mile or kilometer) can equal 1 mile or 1 kilometer on the chart, or you can record minutes walked and let 1 minute equal 1 mile or 1.5 kilometers. Chart your group's progress across a map posted in the facility, and provide incentives for reaching certain landmarks or goals along the way to keep participants excited about their progress. Offer alternative ways for people to participate even if they have difficulty walking. For example, a person who engages in chair exercise or some other physical activity opportunity can record time spent in movement.

Invite the broadest participation by incorporating all dimensions of wellness into the incentive program. For example, 20 minutes spent in any activity designed to improve well-being (e.g., meditation or contemplation stations, stress reduction classes, research on the "travel" destination) can be credited with 20 miles or 20 kilometers. This type of program allows unlimited opportunities for fun activities and celebrations related to the project.

Exercise stations (illustrating specific exercises) can be posted throughout walking courses to add interest and fun. Include a wide range of exercises dealing with range of motion, strength, balance, and coordination. For example, have walkers perform an Achilles stretch (p. 74) or press-back (p. 75) for lower-body exercise. Have them perform a cross-arm (p. 70) or neck stretch (p. 69) for upper-body mobility. The stations can be as simple as line drawings with instructions, but each should identify a specific functional goal. Use handrails where available and the wall by including activities such as wall push-ups and other wall-supported activities (see pp. 82-84 for exercises that can be used in the stations).

Wellness Stations

Using the stations concept, consider ways to address multiple dimensions of well-being. Start with an exercise that promotes an activity of daily living, and then simultaneously address other dimensions of wellness such as emotional, spiritual, social, intellectual, or vocational. Use these stations to encourage contemplation, stimulate intellectual curiosity, promote gratitude, and encourage connections with others. Make sure the physical activity is simple to perform, ensuring success in movement for participants at various levels of functional ability. Look for ways to promote confidence in abilities, self-responsibility, and a positive approach to life's challenges.

Wellness stations can be used as part of class or as an alternative to staff-led programming. Participants can use stations at times that are convenient and at their chosen levels of involvement. Stations offer ongoing opportunities and encouragement for adults to take an active role in maintaining their health and well-being. Refer to chapter 3 for a discussion of the importance of self-responsibility for health outcomes.

Whole-person wellness stations, which I developed in partnership with Jan Montague, clearly illustrate the stations concept. They won a Best Practices Award in 2003 from the National Council on Aging for innovative products meeting the needs of older adults. Some examples of wellness stations are

- *Rise to the Occasion*, illustrated in chapter 3 (figure 3.1, p. 36), addresses the sit-to-stand function (physical) and encourages openness to social interaction and a positive approach to life (social and emotional).

- *Stop and Smell the Roses* invites clients to take the time to enjoy the smallest offerings of joy (emotional) blended with active breathing and upper-body range of motion (physical) (see top right).

- *One Step at a Time* engages participants in a heel-to-toe walk that challenges their balance and posture (physical) and encourages them to see possibilities for improvement rather than focus on limitations (emotional) (see middle right).

- *Count Your Blessings* reminds participants to embrace all the blessings, large or small, in their lives (spiritual and emotional), and it includes a finger-stretching exercise to improve hand function (physical) (see bottom right).

You can use wellness stations individually, incorporate them into other classes, or create a series of stations to provide a unique, highly accessible wellness program. Visit www.kayvannorman.com for further information.

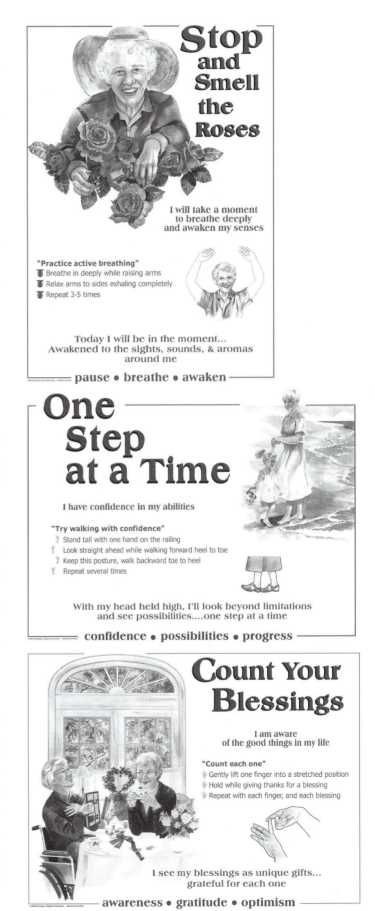

Stop and Smell the Roses

I will take a moment to breathe deeply and awaken my senses

"Practice active breathing"
- Breathe in deeply while raising arms
- Relax arms to sides exhaling completely
- Repeat 3-5 times

Today I will be in the moment... Awakened to the sights, sounds, & aromas around me

pause • breathe • awaken

One Step at a Time

I have confidence in my abilities

"Try walking with confidence"
- Stand tall with one hand on the railing
- Look straight ahead while walking forward heel to toe
- Keep this posture, walk backward toe to heel
- Repeat several times

With my head held high, I'll look beyond limitations and see possibilities....one step at a time

confidence • possibilities • progress

Count Your Blessings

I am aware of the good things in my life

"Count each one"
- Gently lift one finger into a stretched position
- Hold while giving thanks for a blessing
- Repeat with each finger, and each blessing

I see my blessings as unique gifts... grateful for each one

awareness • gratitude • optimism

▷ Wall Exercises

Wall exercises are a useful supplement to chair and chair-supported exercises. Front neutral position is defined as standing facing the wall with both palms on the wall. Side neutral is standing with one side toward the wall, palm on the wall, with the elbow slightly flexed.

▼ **Push-Ups:** Exercisers stand in front neutral position approximately 12 to 15 inches (30-40 centimeters) away from the wall, feet together and palms flat against the wall at shoulder height and shoulder width. They lower themselves toward the wall by bending their elbows and then push away from the wall by straightening the elbows, keeping their palms in contact with the wall, the back straight, and feet flat on the floor while executing the movements slowly (figure 5.17). To create more resistance for improved upper-body strength, participants can perform this exercise with a resistance band placed around the back, one end of the band grasped in each hand. As the exercisers push away from the wall, they also push against the resistance of the stretchy band.

▼ **Wall Crawl:** This exercise begins in front neutral position, very close to the wall with the hands at shoulder level. The exerciser crawls his fingers up the wall reaching to the highest point possible (8 counts) (figure 5.18), and holds for 8 counts. Then he finger-crawls back down the wall (8 counts), steps back away from the wall (hands still in contact), flattens the back, and looks down between his outstretched arms (8 counts). During the sequence, the knees should be slightly flexed and the back as flat as possible.

CAUTION: **Participants with balance difficulties should not perform the second half of the wall-crawl exercise.**

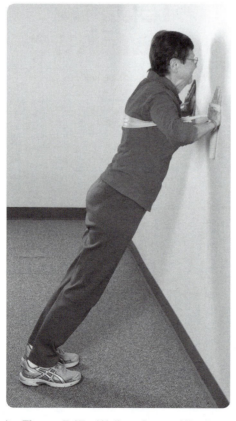

▶ **Figure 5.17** Wall push-up with resistance band.

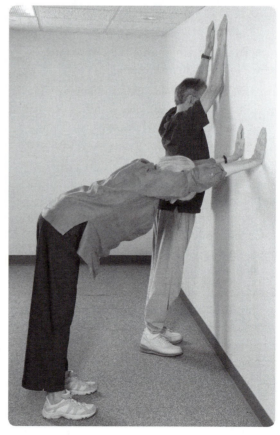

▶ **Figure 5.18** Wall crawl.

▼ **Shoulder Stretch:** Beginning in side neutral position, the exerciser turns slowly away from the wall to look over the opposite shoulder (figure 5.19), holds for 8 counts, and returns slowly to neutral position. She then repeats the movement with the opposite side to the wall.

▼ **Wall Sits:** With the back to the wall and feet approximately 12 to 15 inches (30-40 centimeters) away, the participant flexes the knees until she is in a position similar to sitting in a chair (figure 5.20). (Do not go past 90 degree of flexion.) Then she straightens the knees with the back still against the wall to recover. Exercisers should work up to holding this sitting position for about 15 seconds at a time.

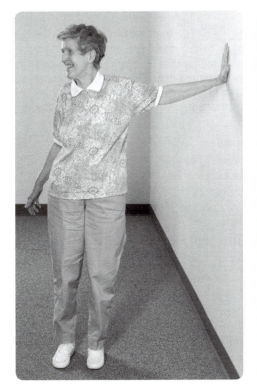

▶ **Figure 5.19** Shoulder stretch.

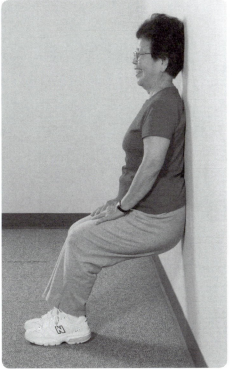

▶ **Figure 5.20** Wall sits.

CAUTION: Do not allow those who are unsteady on their feet, or who have very weak quadriceps muscles, to perform the wall-sit exercise. Do not perform on slick flooring.

■ **Side Leg Lifts:** Beginning in side neutral position, the exerciser does small leg lifts away from the wall (to the side of the body), keeping the toe pointing straight forward (no turnout) and the foot flexed. The supporting leg should also be slightly flexed. Exercisers should do a maximum of 8 consecutive lifts on one side before switching to the other side.

■ **Side Stretch:** Beginning with the left side to the wall, exerciser reaches overhead and continues reaching over to the wall with the right arm (counts 1, 2, 3, 4), bending at the side. She holds the stretch over counts 5, 6, 7, 8 and 1, 2, 3, 4, while breathing normally, and then returns to neutral by bringing the right arm down in front of the body (5, 6, 7, 8). Repeat the stretch 4 times on the right side; then repeat on the left side.

■ **Calf Stretch:** The participant begins in front neutral position with her right toe against the wall and right knee flexed. While extending her left foot back in a wide lunge, keeping the left leg straight (i.e., right forward lunge position), she presses the left heel toward the floor and hold for 8 counts. She then repeats the movement, extending the right foot back.

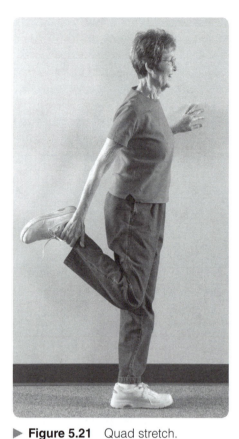

▶ **Figure 5.21**   Quad stretch.

◀ **Quad Stretch:** Beginning with the left side to the wall, the exerciser brings the right heel toward the buttock by flexing the right knee and grasping the right ankle with the right hand (figure 5.21). Hold this stretch, keeping the right knee pointed straight down to the floor and the left knee slightly flexed. Participants should not arch the back, bend at the hip or waist, or move the knee around while stretching.

CAUTION: **The heel should not touch the buttock, because this hyperflexes the knee, placing it in a position vulnerable to injury. The stretch should be repeated on the opposite side. A resistance band or old tie can be looped around the ankle to assist those who are unable to comfortably grasp the ankle.**

■ **Balance:** The exerciser can also do balance work at the wall, rising onto the toes, holding the balance on one foot, or doing small one-leg raises to the front or back. The wall provides a safe support.

Standing Rhythmic Exercises

Standing rhythmic exercise can include simple toe touches and heel presses forward, to the sides, and to the back as well as knee lifts and small kicks, as illustrated on pages 90-91. However, when incorporating these movements into chair exercise classes, consider that some participants may have difficulty with balance. Ensure that participants have support while they perform standing rhythmic exercises, whether using a chair for support, standing next to a wall with one hand on the wall or holding hands in a circle. If exercisers hold hands in a circle during balance activities, be aware of participants' size and strength variations. Make sure that very small participants are not holding hands with considerably larger people, who may pull them off balance during the movements.

LOW-IMPACT AEROBIC EXERCISE

The target audience for this class is the physically independent adult who has enough balance and mobility to move easily from one foot to the other and does not require assistance in walking forward, backward, or sideways. Low-impact aerobic exercise is geared toward improving aerobic endurance through continuous movement to music, with range of motion and coordination mixed in. Other goals include improved strength, flexibility, balance, and agility.

Class Format

Begin the class with a preexercise heart rate check followed by a 10- to 20-minute warm-up of continuous, easy movement to music to increase circulation and help everyone become comfortable with moving. A 20- to 25-minute aerobic phase follows the warm-up and should include careful monitoring of exercise intensity (see chapter 4).

The final phase is a 15- to 20-minute cool-down, including balance and coordination work, and then stretching and relaxation. This is a good time to pass along health information and words of wisdom or humor or to conduct an open forum for sharing thoughts. Schedule class time for socializing, and plan ways to facilitate personal interactions. Some will occur naturally, but you should ensure that the social aspect of class is a priority.

Safe Movement

The main core of the movement should be very simple so that everyone in class is successful in movement most of the time. Complicated combinations and patterns of movement can frustrate many participants and add an element of stress. Always start one body part moving before adding a second. For example, start with a foot movement, and when you can see that all class members are doing the movement correctly, add an arm movement.

To keep the class interesting, use a large variety of arm movements. Movements that use opposing arms and legs alternated with movements that use same-side arms and legs (unison) add variety and improve coordination. Vary your exercise formation, alternating between front-facing rows, circles, lines facing each other, and partners. Many folk dances and simple line dances use movement patterns that can be modified for simplicity and safety. Changes can be as simple as modifying a step–hop to a step–knee lift, adding marching in place between more complex sequences, or changing directions of movement more slowly than in the original dance. For example, a quick slide to the right and left (taking counts *and* 1, and 2-right, *and* 3 and 4-left) can become a hustle step right, then left (taking counts 1 to 4-right, 5 to 8-left). Ferebee-Eckman (2008) offers a variety of folk dance variations that have been field tested in her classes for older adults. See figure 5.2 later in the chapter for a list of common exercises and their most appropriate use in classes.

While designing exercises to add variety and interest, evaluate all movements in terms of the benefits versus the potential risks. For example, movements traveling to the side should not be done until the class has spent adequate time warming up the muscles of the hips and legs by doing toe and heel touches to the front and sides. Side-to-side sliding steps and fast cross-over steps (such as grapevines) pose a high risk of falling and therefore should not be used for group classes that include participants with varying levels of ability. You can modify the grapevine by just stepping to the side, together, and again to the side.

Marching in place is an excellent transition step and should be used between changes of direction or before changes in the movement pattern. This allows everyone to become centered before trying to change directions or focusing on a new series of steps. Face the class (mirror movements) so you can immediately see whether students are having a difficult time with movement. Use hand signals as well as verbal cues while marching in place to indicate to the class the direction in which you intend to travel. When the class is exercising in a circle holding hands and it's time to move to the right, have participants begin tapping the right foot for as many counts as necessary to ensure everyone has the right foot free to step to the side. Return to this tapping whenever necessary to keep people moving in unison in the circle.

Warm-Up and Cool-Down

As discussed in chapter 4, the purpose of the warm-up is to increase body temperature, prepare the body for more vigorous exercise, engage participants socially and emotionally, and observe the body's response to exercise. The purpose of the cool-down is to reduce the body temperature and heart rate to preactivity levels. It is basically the warm-up in reverse with the addition of exercises to increase flexibility and promote relaxation.

Begin your low-impact aerobics classes with 10 to 15 minutes of gentle, continuous movement and easy range of motion activities to slow music (100-110 beats per minute), with a steady and easy-to-distinguish beat. Use easy arm and leg movements that go from small to progressively larger ranges of motion. Begin each sequence with the footwork and then add arm movements. Progressively increase the difficulty of the coordination pattern of the arms. For example, begin with biceps curls and arm swings, front to back and side to side, and one-arm presses front, down, side, and across the body. Progress to two-arm presses to the front, sides, across the body, and overhead, first in unison and then in opposition with the legs. The warm-up is the perfect time to emphasize good posture, proper body mechanics, and breathing techniques during the exercises.

Start the warm-up with simple footwork such as marching in place and toe and heel presses to the front, and then incorporate small kicks and knee lifts to engage the hip more fully before progressing to toe and heel presses and small kicks to the side. Use stationary movement before traveling movement to ensure that participants are transferring weight from foot to foot without balance problems *before* traveling. Start traveling with forward and backward movement, and then progress to step touches side to side before traveling sideways.

Music: "Celestial Soda Pop" and other songs from Deep Breakfast that are 110 to 120 beats per minute

A

March in place (2 counts of 8).

Perform shoulder rolls (forward for 8 counts, backward for 8 counts) while doing slow knee bends.

March again while making a large, slow circle with the arms crossing in front and opening over the head (8 counts).

Keep marching while opening arms to the sides and bringing them back down (2 counts of 8).

B

Alternate toe touches to the front (8 counts).

Repeat while adding arm swings (one arm forward, one arm back—in opposition to footwork) (3 counts of 8).

Repeat A

C

Alternate heel presses to the front (8 counts).

Do heel presses to the front, adding arm swings (one arm forward, one arm back) (3 counts of 8).

Repeat A without the shoulder rolls.

D

Alternate toe touches to the sides (8 counts).

Do toe touches to the sides, adding arm swings side to side in unison.

E

Alternate knee lifts to the front; touch hands to knees (2 counts of 8).

Repeat A without the stationary shoulder rolls.

Repeat B, C, D, and E but replace swinging arms with arms pressing forward, down and up. Use a variety of arm movements in unison and opposition with legs, one arm at a time and both arms together.

F

Alternate small kicks to the front and sides (2 counts of 8).

March in place and perform upper-back squeezes, arm circles, or palm presses diagonally crossing overhead (2 counts of 8).

Alternate small kicks to the front and sides (2 counts of 8).

March in place with arms relaxed.

G

Step right, touch left, step left, touch right (8 counts).

Perform step touches while moving forward (8 counts).

Perform step touches in place (8 counts).

Perform step touches while moving backward (8 counts).

Repeat moving forward and backward (2 counts of 8) while swinging arms side to side in unison.

Perform these sequences and suitable variations for approximately 10 minutes. Use music that is 110 to 120 beats per minute. Begin with a front-facing formation, transition to a circle while holding hands, drop hands and move backward to widen the circle (resume arm movements), and then move back to a front-facing formation or a circle holding hands. Avoid quick, jerky arm movements. Holding hands in a tight circle allows you to perform more intricate foot patterns. You can also use the circle to observe participants' responses to exercise, visit with them, encourage social interaction, and identify a goal for the day.

SAMPLE LOW-IMPACT COOL-DOWN

Music: Max ByGraves, "Somebody Loves Me" medley and other songs that are 110 beats per minute or less

After taking the recovery pulse, begin the cool-down in a circle holding hands.

A

March in place at low intensity (2 counts of 8).

Alternate step touches, moving forward and backward (2 counts of 8).

Drop hands and walk backward for more space—stay in circle formation.

B

Alternate toe touches front (2 counts of 8).

Alternate heel presses front (2 counts of 8).

Alternate toe touches side to side (2 counts of 8) while swinging arms in opposition (keep movements very small).

C

March in place (2 counts of 8).

Perform a large circle with the arms up, over the head, and down (once).

Do shoulder rolls (8 counts forward and 8 counts backward) while bending and straightening the knees.

D

Alternate toe touches side to side (2 counts of 8), arms in opposition.

March in place (8 counts).

Perform toe touches side to side (2 counts of 8), swinging arms in unison.

Repeat, swinging arms gently in opposition and in unison.

Move together to hold hands in circle; tap the right toe in front 8 to 16 times until you can see that all participants have their right foot free to move to the right.

E

Staying in circle, step sideways to the right (step, close, step) for 8 counts.

Repeat stepping to the left (8 counts).

(continued)

SAMPLE LOW-IMPACT COOL-DOWN *(continued)*

Repeat right (1-8) and left (1-8).

Step right (1-4) and step left (5-8).

Repeat right and left (1-8).

Step right (1, 2) and step left (3, 4).

Repeat right (5, 6) and left (7, 8) and again for 8 more counts.

Repeat full sequence.

Note: Cue in advance for the changes in directions. If participants get confused, just march in place and then tap your right toe until everyone has the right foot free to move to the right and begin again. Use music that has a slow, distinct beat of about 110 beats per minute. Stretching music does not need a distinct beat; use relaxing melodies or instrumentals.

Repeat A to D.

Standing in a circle, alternate marching in place while performing standing upper- and lower-body stretches like overhead arm reaches, Achilles stretch (lunge), shoulder stretch (arm crossing in front or back), and hamstring stretch (heel extended to front, flexing forward at hip). Have participants hold hands during the Achilles stretch and hamstring stretch. You can also promote balance by holding hands while lifting the right knee and holding for 4 counts, touching the right toe across the left foot (4 counts), lifting the right knee (4 counts), and stepping onto the right foot. Repeat with the left; then repeat using 2 counts each movement. Limit balance work to very short segments interspersed with stretches. Use this time to connect with participants, talk about what they are going to do after class, and share interesting news.

After 8 to 10 minutes of an active cool-down, check pulses and rating of perceived exertion and then transition to more static flexibility exercises and relaxation exercises. On the mat, perform exercises like low back stretches, hamstring stretches (can use a stretch aid), and straddle stretches. To address abdominal strength, alternate sets of 10 curl-ups between different stretches. End with relaxation breathing; have participants lie on their backs, close their eyes, and take deep breaths. Use quiet instrumental music and visualization of pleasant scenes to enhance relaxation.

Refer to the sidebar (p. 86) for a sample warm-up. Have participants check their heart rates after the warm-up before proceeding to the aerobic phase of class.

Immediately after the aerobic phase, have participants check their heart rate for 10 seconds, walk slowly for 1 minute, and then check their heart rate again for 10 seconds (see chapter 4 for details on checking heart rates). Then begin the cool-down with 5 to 10 minutes of low-intensity, continuous movement to allow the body to transition from exertion to rest. Use small steps side to side and forward and backward, easy marching in place, and heel presses and toe touches to the front and side at progressively lower intensities to return the heart rate and respiration to normal. Keep arm movements small and relaxed, and hold arms predominantly below shoulder level. Mix gentle dynamic stretches and coordination and balance activities in with low-intensity, continuous movement.

The last stage of the cool-down should include static stretches (while the muscles and connective tissue are most pliable) and relaxation activities. Perform stretches on the floor so one muscle group can be isolated for stretching while the rest of the body is relaxed. Devote time at the end of class to relaxation strategies such as deep breathing; play relaxing music and use low lighting if possible. Take time to engage participants socially and emotionally before they leave for the day. Refer to the sidebar for a sample cool-down for healthy older adults.

▶ Specific Aerobic Exercises

The following are descriptions and illustrations of exercise movements that can be used for the warm-up, aerobic, and cool-down phases. During the warm-up phase, exercises are done to slow music (100-110 beats per minute) to increase circulation. Faster and more vigorous movement is done to upbeat music (120-140 beats per minute) during the aerobic phase to elevate the heart rate to the training zone. During the cool-down phase, movements are slow again to bring the heart rate down gradually and prepare the body for stretching. Figure 5.2 lists exercises that can be used in any phase and those that are exclusive to a particular phase.

Low-Impact Land-Based Exercise

Leg movements				Arm movements			
Exercise	**Warm-up**	**Aerobic**	**Cool-down**	**Exercise**	**Warm-up**	**Aerobic**	**Cool-down**
Stationary				One- or two-arm circles (elbow slightly bent)	√	√	
March	√	√	√				
• Toe touch, front	√	√	√	Windshield wipers	√	√	
• Toe touch, side	√	√	√	Biceps curls	√	√	√
• Toe touch, back	√	√	√	Arm swings (opposite side as leg)	√	√	√
• Heel press, forward	√	√	√				
• Heel press, side	√	√	√	Arm swings (same side as leg)	√	√	√
• Small kicks, front	√	√	√				
• Knee lifts	√	√		Arm swings (one arm forward, one backward)	√	√	√
Knee lift, side diagonal	√	√					
Knee lift, small kick (chorus line)	√	√	√	Arm swings (both forward, backward)	√	√	√
Heel lifts to back	√	√	√	Arm waves overhead		√	
Toe touch, forward, side, backward, step	√		√	Palm press, overhead	√	√	
				Palm press, forward	√	√	√
Toe touch, forward, side, forward, step	√		√	Palm press, side	√	√	√
				Palm press, down	√	√	√
Charleston	√	√		Palm press, diagonal overhead	√	√	
Modified box step	√	√					
Side-step touch	√	√	√	Arm crosses	√	√	
Traveling				Front and back crawl		√	
Exercises above marked by asterisk	√	√	√	Scarecrow	√	√	
				Arms scooping	√	√	√
Step, touch (moving forward or backward)	√	√	√	Reach and pull	√	√	√
				Open sides, cross in front	√	√	
Two-step	√	√					
Hustle step, forward	√	√					
Hustle step, backward	√	√		**Transitions:**			
Hustle step, side	√	√		• Always start with one part moving first and then add a second part later. Example: Start moving the feet first, and then add an arm movement.			
Walk or march forward; backward; in your own circle; in large circle while holding hands	√	√	√	• Return to center (marching) before changing directions of movement.			
				• When in circle, give the command "Look right" or (left), "Turn right" or (left), so everyone knows which direction to move.			

▶ **Figure 5.2** Low-impact land-based exercise.

Neutral position is defined as facing forward, standing with weight equally distributed on both feet, and having arms relaxed at the sides. While performing any exercise movement, participants should keep their knees slightly flexed to promote better balance and to ease the transfer of weight from one foot to the other.

Stationary Exercises

- **Marching in Place:** A simple march step (right foot, left foot, right, left) is an excellent transitional movement (or home-base step) to use immediately before changing direction of travel and to return to often. Marching for 8 to 24 counts is appropriate for a transition step.

- ◄ **Heel Presses:** With the weight on the left foot, the exerciser extends her right foot, touches the right heel to the front (count 1) (figure 5.22), brings the right foot back to neutral, and steps on the right foot (2). Then she extends her left foot, touches the left heel to the front (3), brings the left foot back to neutral, and steps on the left foot (4). Repeat the movement: right heel press, step, left heel press, step.

- Heel presses can also be done to the sides. The participant flexes her right foot and extends it at a 45-degree angle to the right (count 1), brings the foot back to neutral and steps on the right foot (2), then extends the left foot at a 45-degree angle to the left side (3), and brings it back to neutral and steps on the left foot (4). Heel presses to the back should not be done.

- ◄ **Toe Touches:** Participants perform the sequence of movement described in the heel presses, but instead of pressing with the heel, they touch the toe out—forward for front toe touch, directly to the side for side toe touches (figure 5.23). Toe touches can be performed to the back.

- ◄ **Small Kicks:** Participants perform the sequence of movement described in the heel press, except instead of pressing with the heel, they give a small kick with the foot and lower leg well below knee height (figure 5.24). Small kicks can be performed to the front or to the side diagonal but should not be attempted to the back.

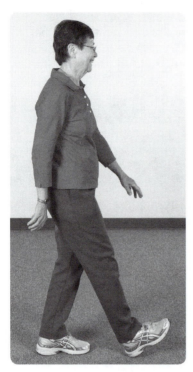

▶ **Figure 5.22** Heel presses.

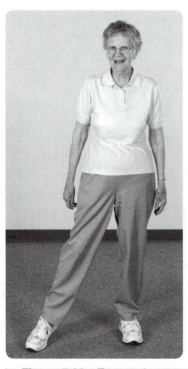

▶ **Figure 5.23** Toe touches.

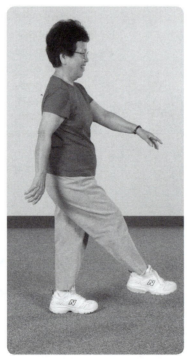

▶ **Figure 5.24** Small kicks.

▶ **Knee Lifts:** With the weight on the left foot, the exerciser lifts the right knee up (count 1) (figure 5.25), steps onto the right foot (2), lifts the left knee up (3), and steps onto the left foot (4), repeating for a set number of repetitions. Knee lifts can be performed to the front or at a 45-degree angle to the side. They can also be performed as doubles; that is, lift right knee (count 1), touch right foot to floor (2), lift right knee again (3), then step on the right foot (4). Do not ask participants to perform knee lifts directly to the side. This requires an advanced degree of hip rotation, which can be unsafe for some adults while standing on one leg.

■ **Chorus Line (knee lift, small kick):** With the weight on the left foot, the participant lifts the right knee (count 1), touches the right toe to the floor next to the left foot (2), gives a small kick with the right foot and lower leg (3), steps on the right foot (4), and then repeats the sequence with the left leg.

▶ **Heel Lifts Back:** With the weight on the left foot, exercisers bend the right knee and lift the right heel toward the buttock (the knee should flex approximately 90 degrees) (figure 5.26) on count 1, step on the right foot (2), lift the left heel toward the buttock (3), and then step on the left foot (4). They should perform this movement with a controlled bending of the knee rather than fling the heel toward the buttock.

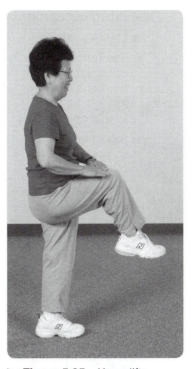

▶ **Figure 5.25** Knee lifts.

■ **Toe Touches Front, Side, Back, and Step:** With the weight on the left foot, the exerciser touches the right toe to the front (count 1), to the right side (2), and to the back (3) and then steps on the right foot next to the left foot (4). He then repeats the sequence with the left foot: touch left foot front (5), to the left (6), and to the back (7) and finally step on the left foot (8). For a simple variation of this movement, the exerciser touches front, side, and front again and then steps.

■ **Charleston:** With the weight on the left foot, the participant gives a small kick forward with the right foot (count 1), steps on the right foot next to the left (2), touches the left foot extended to the back (3), and then steps on the left foot next to the right foot (4). Continue this sequence for a number of repetitions. To perform the exercise on the left side, the participant starts with the weight on the right foot and begins the sequence by kicking forward with the left foot.

■ **Box Step:** With the weight on the left foot, the exerciser steps forward onto the right foot (count 1), forward onto the left foot (2), back onto the right foot (3), and then back onto the left foot (4).

■ **Side Step, Touch:** With the weight on the left foot, participants step to the right side onto the right foot (count 1), touch the left toe next to the right foot (2), step to the left side onto the left foot (3), and then touch the right toe next to the left foot (4).

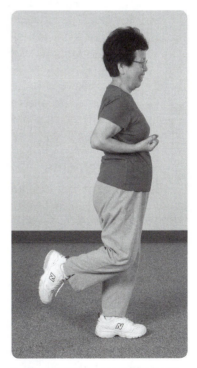

▶ **Figure 5.26** Heel lifts back.

Traveling Movements

- **Marching:** Progress forward or backward with each step.
- **Toe Touches, Heel Presses, and Small Kicks:** Instead of returning the foot to neutral after doing the toe touch, heel press, or small kick (counts 1, 3, 5, 7), participants step forward or backward on counts 2, 4, 6, and 8. For example, touch forward with the right toe (count 1), step forward on right foot (2), touch forward with left toe (3), and step forward with the left foot (4). Toe touches to the back should not travel.
- **Knee Lifts:** Instead of stepping down next to the weight-bearing foot after the knee lift (counts 1, 3, 5, 7), exercisers step forward or backward on counts 2, 4, 6, and 8. Double knee lifts should not travel.
- **Step Touch:** With the weight on the left foot, exercisers step forward onto the right foot (count 1), touch the left toe next to the right foot (2), step forward onto the left foot (3), and touch the right toe next to the left foot (4). This movement can progress backward by having exercisers step backward onto the foot (counts 1 and 3) instead of forward.
- **Two-Step:** (For this exercise, count half beats: 1 *and* 2, 3 *and* 4.) With the weight on the left foot, participants step forward onto the right foot (count 1), step onto the left foot closing next to the right foot (*and*), step forward onto the right foot (2), step forward onto the left foot past the right foot (3), step onto the right foot closing next to the left foot (*and*), and step forward onto the left foot (4). The cueing phrase is "forward right, close, right (1 and 2); forward left, close, left (3 and 4)."
- **Hustle Step:** Beginning with the weight on the left foot, exercisers travel forward, stepping right (count 1), left (2), right (3), and touch the left toe next to the right foot (4). They repeat the movement but travel backward by stepping back onto the left foot (5), right foot (6), and left foot (7) and touch the right toe next to the left foot (8). The cueing phrase is "forward right, left, right, tap left; backward left, right, left, tap right."
- **Hustle Step Side:** With the weight on the left foot, exercisers step right onto the right foot (count 1), bring the left foot next to the right and step on the left foot (2), step to the right side again onto the right foot (3), and then touch the left toe next to the right foot (4). They repeat the sequence but travel to the left by stepping left (5), close right next to left (6), step to left (7), and touch with the right toe (8). The cueing phrase is "side right, close, right, tap left; side left, close, left, tap right."

Arm Movements

Start with a foot movement or pattern, and when you can see that all class members are doing it correctly, add an arm movement. The neutral position is arms hanging down in a relaxed position next to the sides of the body.

- **Arm Circles:** Exercisers circle one or both arms to the front or out to the sides, keeping the elbows slightly bent throughout the motion.
- **Windshield Wipers:** With both arms in front of the body, elbows flexed, palms turned forward, participants sweep both arms to the right and then to the left, mimicking the action of windshield wipers.
- **Biceps Curls:** Exercisers extend both arms down in front of the body with palms facing up. They flex the right elbow (palm up), and then while straightening the right elbow, flex the left elbow (palm up). Repeat the motion with the cues "flex the right, left, right, left." Curls may also be done with both arms simultaneously and with 1- to 3-pound (.5- to 1.5-kilogram) weights.
- **Arm Swings:** Participants swing one or both arms to the side, forward, or backward. Arm swings can be done in unison (i.e., same-side leg and arm) (figure 5.27*a*) to the leg work or in opposition (figure 5.27*b*). The swings can also be done with one arm swinging forward while the other arm swings back, either in opposition or in unison with the leg work. Allow 2 counts for each swing in any direction.

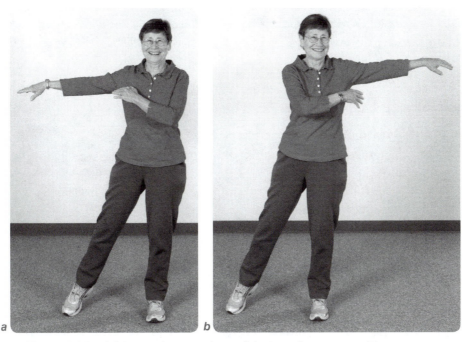

▶ **Figure 5.27** *(a)* Arm swings—unison; *(b)* arm swings—opposition.

- **Arm Waves Overhead:** With the arms extended over the head, palms facing out, participants sway with both arms right, left, right, left. This can also be done with one arm extended overhead.

▶ **Palm Presses:** Beginning in neutral position, exercisers flex one or both elbows, bringing the hands toward the shoulders, and then extend the elbows by pressing out with the wrists flexed and palms turned straight up (palm press up), to the front (palm press forward), to the sides (palm press open to sides), or straight down (palm press down). This can also be done with one arm at a time pressing up, forward, side, down, or at a diagonal (figure 5.28), crossing overhead.

- **Arm Crosses:** Beginning in neutral position, participants cross both arms in front of the body at hip level, open to sides, then cross both arms behind the body (hip level), and open to sides (1 count for each movement). Front arm crosses can also be done at chest level, alternating right over left, then left over right. The elbows should be slightly bent.

- **Scarecrow:** Beginning in neutral position, exercisers lift the bent elbows out to the sides, palms facing backward, and then straighten the arms to the sides by extending the elbows while keeping the palms facing backward. They continue the movement, flexing and extending the elbows.

- **Open Sides, Cross Front:** Beginning in neutral position, exercisers open arms wide to the sides (2 counts) and then cross arms in front of the body at chest height (2 counts).

- **Arm Scoops:** With the elbows bend and hands next to hips, participants scoop the arms in a small circle at hip level.

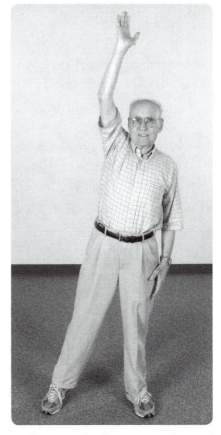

▶ **Figure 5.28** Palm press diagonal.

- **Reach and Pull:** Beginning in neutral position, exercisers reach both arms straight forward at chest level and then pull elbows back to hip level, using 1 count for each movement.

- See the sidebar for an example of a low-impact aerobic phase.

SAMPLE LOW-IMPACT AEROBICS PHASE

Music: "Chattanooga Choo-Choo Boy" and "In the Mood" (Glen Miller), "England Swings" (Roger Miller), "Bye Bye Blackbird" (Max Bygraves), and other songs with 120 to 140 beats per minute

A

Do the hustle step forward (8 counts) and backward (8 counts).

Do the hustle step forward (4 counts) and backward (4 counts); repeat.

March in place (8 counts).

In place, kick to the front and swing arms in opposition (8 counts), kick to the side swinging both arms in unison (8 counts), repeat.

March in place (8 counts).
Repeat sequence A.

B

Do the hustle step to the right side (8 counts) with arm scoops, march in place (8 counts), and repeat to the left.

Repeat using 4 counts each right, marching, left, marching.

Do the hustle step to the right side (8 counts) and left side (8 counts) while pushing arms overhead.

March in place (8 counts).

Repeat using 4 counts each right, left, right, left.

March in place (16 counts).
Repeat sequence B.

C

Stand in place and do knee lifts while swinging arms in opposition (8 counts).

Do side knee lifts, elbows to knees (8 counts).

While moving forward, do knee lifts (8 counts), touching each knee with both hands.

Do side knee lifts in place, elbows to knees (8 counts).

March in place (8 counts).

While moving backward, do knee lifts, touching each knee with both hands.

March in place (16 counts) while reaching arms overhead and into a big circle.
Repeat C.

D

The group does step touches while moving into a circle (16-24 counts); arms swing in unison until participants are close enough to join hands.

Perform kicks moving forward (8 counts) and then backward (8 counts), holding hands.

Perform kicks moving forward (8 counts), and then release hands and move backward (8-16 counts) to form a very large open circle while arms swing in opposition.

Do the hustle step forward into circle (4 counts) and then backward (4 counts); repeat.

March in place (8 counts) and then march backward (8 counts).
Repeat D but finish the sequence by marching back into front-facing position.

E

Do heel lifts to the back while arms reach and pull (2 counts of 8).

Perform a knee lift and small kick, alternating legs (2 counts of 8).

March in place (8 counts).

Do toe touches to the front (8 counts) and heel presses to the front (8 counts) while arms open to the side and cross in front.

Perform knee lifts (8 counts) while pressing palms overhead.

March in place (8 counts).

Repeat E.

F

Perform step touches while moving into two lines facing each other; march in place to identify partner in opposite line (16-24 counts).

Hustle step forward (4 counts) toward partner, and then hustle step backward (4 counts); repeat.

Walk forward around partner and then backward to starting place (do-se-do) (8 counts); repeat in other direction.

Repeat hustle step and do-se-do sequence.

March in place (8 counts).

Do heel presses forward (8 counts), heel presses side (8 counts), small kicks forward (8 counts, and small kicks sideways (8 counts); with the arms, alternate pressing palms up, down, and side to side.

Repeat F from hustle steps.

Repeat entire sequence from A to F either in the same order or in random order, or use any combination of the segments. Vary the arm movements, vary the formations, and increase or decrease the number of repetitions. Keep all arm movements at a comfortable speed. For example, "arms open to the side and cross in front" would use 2 counts for arms opening and 2 counts for arms crossing rather than 1 count opening and 1 count crossing. Alternate slower aerobic music (beats per minute in the 120s) with faster aerobic music (130s-140s), and remember to check the pulse rate at least three times during the aerobics phase. Check 1-minute and recovery pulse rates at the end of the aerobics session (see chapter 4). Visit the author's Web site, www .kayvannorman.com, for videos demonstrating the full sequences.

Floor Exercises

Floor exercises should always be done on a mat or other soft surface. If your facility does not provide large mats, class members must provide their own; fortunately, there are many different kinds of affordable individual exercise mats. If you have a participant who is unable or unwilling to go to the floor for stretches, you can modify some exercises to be done in a chair or against the wall.

- **Curl-Ups:** Lying in neutral back position (i.e., on the back, feet flat on the floor, knees flexed) with hands either behind the neck (not on the head) or crossed in front of the chest, the exerciser performs slow, small curl-ups bringing the shoulders no more than 6 inches (15 centimeters) off the floor. To avoid neck strain, do a maximum of 10 repetitions at a time and alternate curl-ups with hamstring stretches, hip tucks, or other floor work that puts the neck in a totally relaxed position.

- **Knee Hugs:** Beginning in neutral back position, participants wrap their arms under their knees and bring the knees slowly to the chest, holding to gently stretch the low back while breathing normally. Hold for 12 to 16 counts.

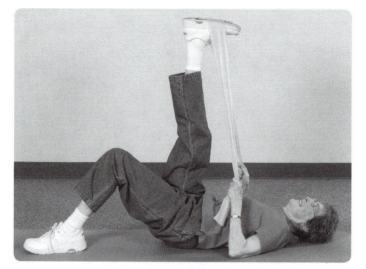

▶ **Figure 5.29** Hamstring stretch.

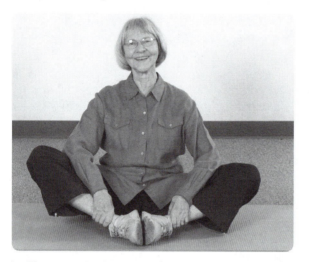

▶ **Figure 5.30** Frog sit.

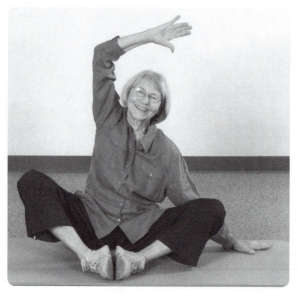

▶ **Figure 5.31** Frog sit with side reach.

◀ **Hamstring Stretch:** From neutral back position, exercisers extend the right knee so the right leg points straight up with the foot flexed and hold the leg in this position to stretch the right hamstring (figure 5.29). A resistance band, an old tie, or a strip of fabric can be used to assist in this stretch. Wrap the aid around the sole of the foot and use it to help keep the leg in a stretched position. Repeat the stretch on the left side. This exercise can also be done sitting on the floor with the legs extended to the front and using a resistance band for a stretch aide.

◀ **Frog Sit:** Participants sit with knees out to the sides and the soles of the feet together. They place the elbows on the knees and gently push down to stretch the muscles of the inner thighs (figure 5.30).

◀ **Frog Sit With Side Reach:** Beginning in frog-sit position, exercisers place the left hand on the floor next to the left leg and gently drop over to the left side, stretching the muscles on the right side of the body. Then they repeat the stretch to the right side. A more advanced stretch is to reach the right arm up and over the head toward the left (figure 5.31).

▶ **Straddle Stretch:** Participants sit straight up with their legs extended open to the sides. Keeping the back and the legs straight, they slowly flex forward at the hips until they feel a stretch in the hamstring and hip extensor muscles (figure 5.32). Hold the stretch for 8 to 16 counts. If participants feel a stretch just by getting into the beginning position, have them place their hands on the floor behind their buttocks to help keep their back and the legs straight.

▶ **Low Back Stretch:** Lying on their backs with the legs extended straight out on the mat, exercisers bend the right knee, place the right foot next to the left knee, and then gently allow the right knee to cross over the top of the left leg while trying to keep both shoulders on the floor (figure 5.33). Hold the stretch for 12 to 24 counts, reminding participants to breathe normally. Repeat the stretch to the right side.

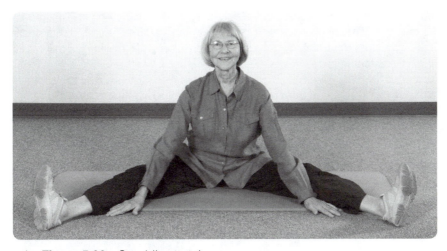

▶ **Figure 5.32** Straddle stretch.

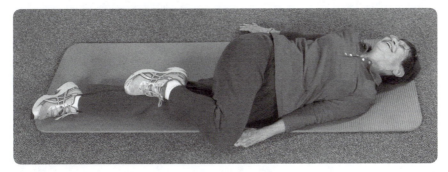

▶ **Figure 5.33** Low back stretch.

- **Side Leg Lift:** Lying on the left side with the hips in a line perpendicular to the floor, feet pointing forward (i.e., no turnout at hip) and the ankles flexed, exercisers do small lifts with the right leg (8-16 repetitions). They do *not* prop the head up with the left hand but rather keep the left arm extended flat on the mat with the head resting on the arm. Then they repeat the exercise lying on the right.

▼ **Modified Push-Up:** Participants begin by lying face down on the mat with both palms next to the shoulders. Slowly, they raise the body from the mat by pushing with the hands and extending the elbows while keeping the knees and feet on the mat. With the back straight and the head in line with the neck and back, participants lower themselves down until the chest almost touches the mat and then push up again, fully extending the elbows (figure 5.34). If some of your participants lack the strength to do the push-up, have them begin in an elbows-extended position and lower themselves to the mat.

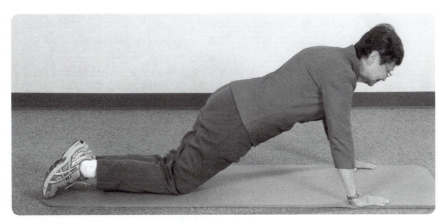

▶ **Figure 5.34** Modified push-up.

▼ **Hip Tuck:** Lying in the neutral back position, exercisers tuck the hips upward by contracting the lower abdominal muscles and buttocks (figure 5.35). They hold this position for 4 to 8 counts and then return to the neutral back position. This is a very small movement during which participants should keep the back in contact with the floor.

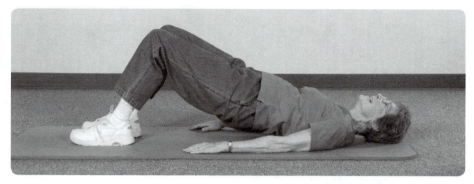

▶ **Figure 5.35** Hip tuck.

■ **Cat Arch:** Beginning with hands and knees on the mat, participants arch their backs (like an angry cat), hold, and then release to the beginning position.

▼ **Low Back Strength:** Exercisers lie face down on the mat with their elbows and lower arms flat, palms down. They slowly raise the upper body off the mat 6 to 8 inches (15-20 centimeters) (figure 5.36), hold (4-8 counts), and return to beginning position. Exercisers should keep the neck in line with the back (look at floor) and avoid pushing with the arms. The back should do the work while the arms provide balance and support.

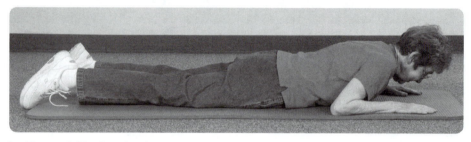

▶ **Figure 5.36** Low back strength.

Note: Wall exercises can be used in place of or in conjunction with floor exercises to promote strength and flexibility. Some participants are uncomfortable doing floor exercises and prefer working against the wall. All of the wall exercises described at the beginning of this chapter can be used in the cool-down phase of a low-impact aerobics class (see pp. 82-84 for exercise descriptions).

▶ Balance and Coordination

For balance activities, have the participants stand next to a wall, in the center of the floor in lines holding hands, or in a circle holding hands. Use balance activities during the cool-down only.

CAUTION: Participants with osteoporosis should refrain from standing on one leg for more than 8 counts at a time. People who are in the later stages of osteoporosis should avoid exercising while standing on one leg.

■ **Leg Lift:** Exercisers do small straight-leg lifts (approximately 6 inches [15 centimeters] off the floor) to the front or to the front diagonal. Hold for a maximum of 12 counts before changing to the other leg.

■ **Knee Lift:** Participants lift one knee to the front at a 90-degree angle and hold for a maximum of 12 counts.

▶ **Knee Lift With Cross:** With the weight on the left leg, exercisers lift the right knee to center (count 1), cross the right leg over the left leg and touch the right toe to the left of the left foot (figure 5.37) (2), lift the right knee back to center (3), and then step onto the right foot (4). They repeat the movement crossing left leg over right.

■ **Rise Up:** Standing next to a wall, or in lines or circles holding hands, participants rise up onto their toes and balance for 8 counts, return their heels to the floor, and then bend their knees (keeping the heels on the floor). They repeat the sequence 3 to 6 times.

■ **Toe Tap:** Standing in a circle holding hands, exercisers extend the right leg to the front and tap the right toe to the floor, using the ankle to flex and tap the toe. They tap 1, 2, 3, 4, 5, 6, 7, step onto the right foot (8), repeat with the left foot tapping 7 counts, and then step onto the left foot (8). You

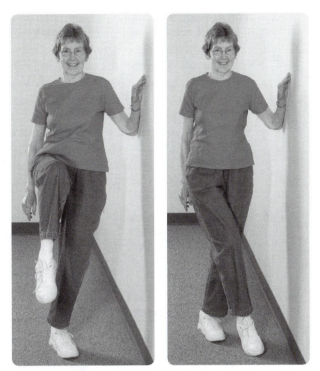

▶ **Figure 5.37** Knee lift with cross.

may repeat the sequence using a countdown of 4 taps, then 2 taps, and 1 tap on each foot.

■ **Side Step Sequence:** Standing in a circle holding hands, exercisers step to the right onto the right foot (1), step the left foot next to the right (2), step to the right on the right foot (3), and tap with the left foot beside the right foot (4). They repeat the sequence traveling to the left (5, 6, 7, 8), ending with a tap with the right foot. Then they step to the right with the right foot (1), tap with the left foot beside the right foot (2), step to the left with the left foot (3), tap with the right foot beside the left foot (4), and repeat the movement to the right, tap, left, tap, for counts 5, 6, 7, and 8. Cue the sequence, "Step right, close, right, tap left; step left, close, left, tap right; step right, tap, step left, tap, step right, tap, step left, tap."

▶ Social Interaction

Use a variety of formations to facilitate social interaction throughout the entire class period. For example, a large circle with participants holding hands for parts of the warm-up, aerobics, and cool-down allows everyone to see each other, exchange smiles, and even talk a little (especially good for the cool-down phase). Arranging participants in two lines facing each other also allows exchanges between class members and makes a good transition to partner work. Develop activities that are specifically designed to foster interaction.

▶ **Shoulder Rub:** Have the participants find partners who are approximately the same height. One of the partners stands behind the other and gives him or her a shoulder rubdown; then they switch places (figure 5.38). This can also be done in a small circle.

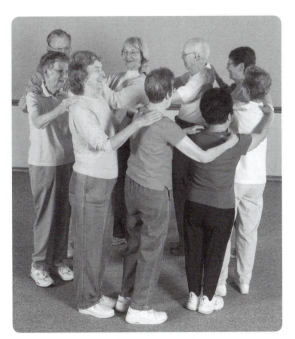

▶ **Figure 5.38** Circle shoulder rub.

- **Writing Names:** With partners, one person stands behind the other and writes the other's name on her or his back; then they switch places. Instruct students to state their full name to their partners (even if they have known them for years). This is a great way to help participants learn and recall each other's names, and it feels great!
- **Ball Toss:** Have participants form a circle. Begin by calling out your own name and handing a ball to the person next to you. The rest of the people in the circle repeat your name in unison. The ball continues around the circle as each person calls out his or her name, everyone repeats the name, and the person passes the ball to the next person. After one time around the circle, the last person holding the ball calls out a name of anyone around the circle and tosses the ball to that person. This is a fun activity that helps people remember names and improves eye–hand coordination. Either a large rubber ball or a small Koosh ball is a good choice for this activity.
- **Sharing Time:** Share a thought for the day, a poem, a funny anecdote, health tips, or something that is happening in your life, and encourage class members to do the same. When this becomes a regular part of your class, people will frequently bring items to share.

RESISTANCE TRAINING EXERCISE

Resistance training prevents and reverses the loss of muscle mass, strength, and power typically associated with aging. It also improves bone density and mass and reduces risk factors for numerous chronic diseases. When done properly, resistance training is a safe and effective strategy to help adults retain or regain functional independence, self-efficacy, and a positive quality of life. This section explains principles of resistance training, outlines appropriate training protocols for strength and power, discusses resistance training equipment, and provides specific exercises focused on maintaining and improving functional ability.

Regular participation in many physical activities improves muscular strength, power, and endurance, but for significant strength and power gains exercise must be done against resistance. Progressive resistance training (PRT), which involves gradually increasing the level of resistance as a participant becomes stronger, has been proven safe and effective for all levels of functional ability. Fiatarone's (1994) research with 100 frail nursing home residents aged 72 to 98 proved that even physically dependent older adults with multiple chronic conditions could benefit from high-intensity progressive resistance training. The proper intensity is key to improvement. Prior researchers had used low-intensity strength training (40-60% 1RM) and had concluded that older adults could not improve strength. Fiatarone's subjects trained at the intensity of 80% of a 1-repetition maximum (1RM), which means training with a resistance equal to 80% of the maximum amount of resistance a person can lift one time. For example, if a person can lift a maximum of 10 pounds (4.5 kilograms) one time in good form, then she would train with 8 pounds (3.6 kilograms).

Resistance training includes training for strength, defined as the amount of force a muscle can generate, and training for power, defined as the ability to generate force quickly. Power training requires high-velocity contractions, which means contracting the muscles quickly against resistance. Research shows that muscle power is lost at a much faster rate (3.5% per year) than strength alone and is also more closely associated with performance of the activities of daily living (Foldvari et al., 2000). In addition, power training (high-velocity training) is more effective than strength training for improving physical function (Hazell et al., 2007). See chapter 4 (p. 62) for a discussion of how power affects functional ability.

Resistance work can be performed using equipment such as resistance bands, hand and ankle weights, and medicine balls or by using body weight as the resistance (as in push-ups) and exercising in water. However, using resistance training machines has the most potential to significantly improve functional ability.

To train power, equipment and movement strategies must safely allow speed of movement. This poses a problem when trying to train power with the most common type of resistance machines, iron weight stack equipment. The standard training protocol for weight stack equipment requires a 3-second lift to control the momentum of the weight stack, effectively negating the speed component. Equipment selection can have a significant impact on the success of resistance training programs for older adults. Refer to the sidebar for a checklist to help you evaluate equipment conducive to training both strength and power.

EQUIPMENT CHECKLIST

▶ Is nonintimidating in appearance and function

▶ Is user-friendly, simple, and easy to operate

▶ Allows high-velocity movement (power training)

▶ Is easy to enter and exit by people with a variety of functional abilities and disabilities

▶ Has a very low starting resistance (0-2 pounds [0-1 kilogram])

▶ Can accommodate very small increments of resistance (1-2 pounds [.5-1 kilogram])

▶ Provides low-impact resistance

▶ Clearly indicates where to sit and where to place hands and feet

▶ Provides adjustments that allow people of various body sizes (minimum height 4 feet 10 inches [148 centimeters]) and those with functional limitations to be in the proper position while exercising

▶ Has easily adjustable hand, seat, and pad positions

▶ Allows user to change resistance from a seated position

▶ Provides instructional placards with simple diagrams and text in a font that is easy to read

▶ Provides range of motion limiters to accommodate joint dysfunction

▶ Is made by a manufacturer that has a demonstrated track record and that provides high-quality product, workmanship, service, and training

Avoid multistation resistance machines that promise a full-body workout with one piece of equipment. They are often confusing to operate and sacrifice adjustment options to gain the multifunction approach.

Principles of Strength Training

This information is designed to provide resistance training principles appropriate for older adults. These are basic guidelines and should not be used as a substitute for proper supervision. Qualified personnel should supervise strength training programs to ensure proper exercise form, intensity, and duration. It is important to understand the following basic definitions:

- **Concentric contraction:** a muscle-shortening contraction. For example, the biceps muscle exhibits a concentric contraction as the elbow flexes during a biceps curl.

- **Duration:** the length of time spent in an exercise session.

- **Eccentric contraction:** a muscle-lengthening contraction, usually occurring against the pull of gravity. For example, when extending the elbow after a biceps curl, the biceps muscle has to contract eccentrically to control the

speed and force of the extension; otherwise the forearm would simply drop open rapidly.

- **Frequency:** how often the strength training sessions are performed (e.g., 2 times per week).

- **Intensity:** a measure of how much effort is used during the exercises.

- **1-repetition maximum (1RM):** the maximum amount of weight a person can correctly lift one time (i.e., 1 repetition).

- **Power:** the amount of force a muscle can generate quickly.

- **Progressive overload principle:** principle that states a muscle will become stronger only if it is subjected to a workload that is greater than what has been previously used. Therefore, progressive resistance training (PRT) applies this principle.

- **Range of motion:** the degree of angle a joint can move through considering the joint itself and the length of the muscles, tendons, and ligaments attached to the joint.

- **Repetition:** completion of one exercise (e.g., lift and return) with the designated resistance.

- **Resistance:** the amount of force that is being worked against, often referred to as to the amount of weight lifted.

- **Sets:** the number of times a specific exercise is performed (i.e., repetitions). For example, at the proper intensity for strength gains, 8 to 12 repetitions of an exercise can be performed before fatigue occurs or form is compromised. Therefore, 8 to 12 repetitions are referred to as 1 set of that specific exercise.

- **Strength:** the amount of force a muscle can generate.

Strength Training Protocols

To ensure safe and effective programming, you must observe strength training protocols including proper intensity, frequency, duration, and techniques.

- **Intensity:** Strength training should be performed at about 80% of a person's 1RM. Have students begin with a weight they can lift correctly 8 times. When 12 repetitions can be performed with proper form, increase resistance by 5% to 10% and begin again with 8 repetitions.

- **Frequency:** Strength training should be performed two or three nonconsecutive days per week. Allow at least 1 day of rest between training sessions so the body can rebuild muscle tissue.

- **Duration:** The time spent in each training session is determined by the number of exercises, repetitions, and sets performed.

- **Number of exercises:** A minimum of one exercise per major muscle group should be performed.

- **Repetitions:** An exercise should be performed 8 to 12 times in most cases. This number is determined by initial fitness level, goals, and contraindications.

- **Sets:** Two or three sets are the standard number for improving strength; however, the number of sets performed is determined by initial fitness level, goals, and contraindi-

cations. Research indicates that 1 set at the proper intensity (80% of 1RM) can provide very similar gains in strength as 2 or 3 sets. For general conditioning, 1 or 2 sets are appropriate.

- **Technique:** To ensure safety and effectiveness of strength training, proper technique should be used at all times, including the following:

  - **Proper adjustments:** Ensure that students use the proper seat, range of motion, and leg and arm pad adjustments to fit body size and ensure proper body mechanics. For exercises that rotate around a single joint, the middle of the joint should be at the pivot point of the machine. For example, when a participant is seated in the leg extension machine, the pivot point of the machine (mechanism that allows extension and flexion) should line up directly with the center of the knee joint.

  - **Range of motion:** Full ROM should be the goal for all exercises when possible; however, exercises should be performed through the pain-free range of motion only.

  - **Breathing patterns:** Continuous, natural breathing patterns should be used while training. Remind students to avoid the Valsalva maneuver (holding their breath to exert more force) or any prolonged holding of breath. In general, students should breathe out on the exertion phase of the exercise.

  - **Speed of movement:** Iron weight stack equipment requires taking 2 or 3 seconds to move or "lift" the weight to overcome the forces created by momentum. Some types of resistance equipment do not require controlling the speed. *Note:* To train power, equipment must allow the speed component (refer to the sidebar checklist).

Power Training Protocols

Power training protocols are very similar to strength training protocols. The differences are as follows:

- **Speed of movement:** Power training requires high-velocity (rapid) movement. For example, instead of taking 3 seconds to move the weight, the concentric phase (contraction) should happen as quickly as possible. The eccentric phase is done more slowly (2-3 seconds). Do not attempt power training protocols with iron weight stack equipment.

■ **Intensity:** Research is still being conducted on the optimal intensity for power training: 50% to 70% seems to be the standard range being tested. I use 60% of 1RM to train power. Take the time to read Hazell and colleagues' (2007) review of research on the topic, and keep abreast of new research by reading the *Journal of Aging and Physical Activity*. Most of the power training research conducted to date with older adults has used Keiser pneumatic equipment; see the research link on this company's Web site at www.keiser.com/kioa/.

If you have any influence on the type of equipment purchased for an adult resistance training program, use the equipment checklist (see sidebar) and advocate for equipment that facilitates speed of movement, such as pneumatic, magnetic, and hydraulic equipment. Share research on how power affects function to make your case with decision makers. Carefully evaluate the pros and cons of hydraulic and magnetic resistance equipment, which can train power but requires concentric contractions through the entire exercise (i.e., users must push against resistance and then pull against resistance to return to beginning position). This eliminates training of the eccentric or muscle-lengthening contraction that has been proven important to tasks like lowering oneself onto a chair. Training power without machines is a little more challenging but can be done with medicine balls, resistance bands, water resistance, and even body weight. Over the next decade, strategies for training power with and without equipment will gain a great deal more attention. See pages 108-111 for specific exercises using just body weight and speed of movement to train power.

Program Basics

A resistance training program focused on promoting functional independence can be accomplished using six to eight machines that address the large muscle groups. Just because there are 15 machines in a room doesn't mean it is necessary or optimal to use them all. Once the major muscle groups are exercised (chest, upper back, legs, buttocks), extra exercises must be chosen carefully to correct muscle imbalances and provide additional work on areas critical to function; otherwise, any extra exercises can just add more time to the session without much benefit or can even exacerbate problems.

Movement That Matters

It is common for adults to have shorter, stronger chest muscles and longer, weaker upper-back muscles resulting from repetitive movement patterns. Consider the typical activities in a day and how many times the chest muscles contract (and shorten) while one is working at a computer, performing household duties, driving, or even walking if the person isn't conscious of good posture. Compare that with the number of times the average person performs movements that contract and shorten the upper-back muscles, which requires pulling the shoulder blades together in back. Therefore, performing an exercise like the seated butterfly, which isolates and strengthens the chest muscles, would not be a priority, especially given that chest muscles are already addressed through the chest press. Time would be better spent on stretching the chest muscles and strengthening the upper back.

Some degrees of shoulder, knee, neck, or back problems are common among adults, which could put them at risk for injury. Frequently remind participants to only train through the pain-free range of motion; as with all exercise programs, identify movement that matters and weigh the benefits against the potential risks for all movement choices.

Proper Body Mechanics

Ensure that participants are exercising on equipment that allows adjustments for body size. This is one reason to avoid the all-in-one multifunction machines. It is often tempting to purchase these machines because they generally cost less than individual machines and can fit into smaller spaces, and it sounds great to have all the exercises you need in one machine. However, if you use the equipment checklist in the sidebar (p. 101) to evaluate multifunction machines, you can see where they fall short in many areas. For example, most multifunction machines are designed with 6-foot (1.8-meter) male athletes in mind and provide few adjustments for different body sizes. These machines usually fail to accommodate an average older adult woman and many smaller men, forcing many people to exercise against resistance in positions that put them at risk for muscle and joint injury. Because these machines are difficult to adjust and operate, it is very common to see them sitting in the corner of the room with no one going near them. This forms an active barrier to resistance training participation, especially for adults in the precontemplation, contemplation, and preparation stages of change.

Special Concerns

Some exercises like the knee extension are great for leg strength but can pose a problem for participants with knee problems. An orthopedic surgeon once told me that he would like to remove knee extension machines from all gyms because they are so often used improperly! To safely use the knee extension machine, ensure that the pivot point of the machine matches the center of the knee joint and make sure participants begin the exercise with the knee flexed at 90 degrees. Many machines have ROM adjustments that start with the knee flexed past 90 degrees. This places a great deal of unnecessary stress on the knee joint, so encourage participants to double-check the adjustment before starting the exercise. Participants with knee problems can avoid the knee extension machine and instead use the leg press machine, which works all the lower-body muscles.

The seated butterfly machine can pose a problem for participants with shoulder problems. Butterfly machines that do not have range of motion limiters often place the shoulder joints in a hyperextended position at the beginning of the exercise, making them more vulnerable to injury.

In short, take the time to evaluate which muscles each machine targets and determine the benefits versus the risks for that exercise. Choose machines that allow proper adjustments and target functional movement. Remember that more is not always better and that exercises isolating a very specific muscle group (like a biceps curl) are often not the best use of participants' time.

Proper Intensity

The proper intensity for strength training is generally 80% of 1RM, which translates to a weight that can be lifted a minimum of 8 times. If a participant can easily lift the weight 12 to 14 times, then increase the resistance 5% to 10% and begin again with 8 repetitions. This ensures the resistance is progressive, that is, it increases as strength increases.

Determining a participant's exact 1RM for strength training requires a 1RM test. Carefully instruct participants on the purpose of a 1RM test and ensure they use proper technique while testing. The following is a standard protocol for finding the 1RM for strength.

Step 1: Warm-up (general)

Do 5 to 10 minutes of low-intensity cardiovascular work using a cardio machine or continuous low-intensity movement.

Step 2: Familiarization

1. Describe the 1RM test and explain rating of perceived exertion (RPE) (see p. 59).
2. Demonstrate the individual exercise, noting correct form, full range of motion, and correct breathing.
3. Adjust equipment positions for client and record them on a form.
4. Have client perform 2 repetitions using *minimal* resistance (this should be very easy).
5. Check for correct technique (repeat steps 1-3 if necessary).

Step 3: Warm-up (specific) and test

1. Select warm-up resistance, which should again be very easy.
2. Perform 5 repetitions.
3. Evaluate difficulty on a scale of 1 to 5 and adjust weight to approximate the client's likely 1RM.
4. Allow 30 seconds between trials.
5. Repeat test sequence until subject can no longer complete 1 repetition with correct form through a full range of motion.
6. Record the 1RM value.

▶ Specific Resistance Training Exercises

The following resistance training circuit alternates upper- and lower-body exercises to maximize effectiveness and minimize fatigue. This circuit can be performed after a cardiovascular training program. If aerobics do not precede the resistance training, have participants warm up for at least 10 minutes by performing low-intensity, continuous movements that increase body temperature and (when possible) mimic the range of motion participants will use during strength training.

Go through the entire circuit (the following eight exercises) a minimum of one time at the appropriate intensity (80% 1RM for strength training, 60% 1RM for power training). Make sure participants are performing the proper speed of movement as well. If they are using weight stack equipment, each concentric phase should take 2 or 3 seconds. If they are using pneumatic, hydraulic, or magnetic equipment, then they are not restricted by momentum and so can move more quickly. If participants are training power (not on iron weight stacks), they should move as fast as possible on the concentric phase. Only train power on equipment designed for high-speed movement or with body weight as described on pages 108-111. A second set of these exercises can also be performed if desired, or participants can repeat some of the exercises.

If you have access to a limited number of machines or are restricted by time, focus on machines that train large muscle groups, like the leg press for the lower body and the chest press, upper-back machine, lat pull, or shoulder press for the upper body. Instruct participants to stretch after training to maintain joint mobility and range of motion, giving special attention to the muscles and joints engaged in the resistance training.

▼ **Upper Back:** This machine exercises the whole upper back including the trapezius, deltoid, latissimus dorsi, rhomboids, biceps, and triceps. This exercise contributes to upright posture, proper back alignment, and muscle balance. Make adjustments so the desired handgrips are lined up just above the shoulders and just at the extended reach. Have participants pull their elbows back smoothly while simultaneously sitting upright on the first repetition (figure 5.39) and then maintain the upright posture through the remaining repetitions.

▼ **Leg Press:** This machine exercises the largest muscle groups in the body—quadriceps, hamstrings and gluteals—while allowing the upper body to rest. The leg press exercise improves balance and contributes to walking, rising from sitting to standing, and lowering from standing to sitting. The participant places the feet in the middle of the foot plate and begins with the knees close to the chest and feet in alignment with the knees (not turning out or in). The participant should extend the legs fully *without locking the knees* (figure 5.40) and then smoothly return to the beginning position.

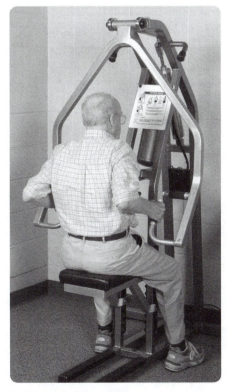 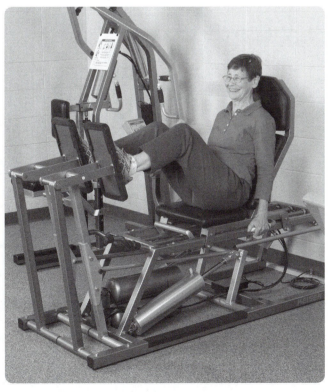

▶ **Figure 5.39** Upper-back exercise. ▶ **Figure 5.40** Leg press.

◀ **Seated Chest Press:** This machine exercises the chest muscles (pectorals) and the triceps and trains the muscles that contribute to lifting and carrying. Adjust the seat height so handgrips are just below the shoulders. Have the participant smoothly extend her arms forward (figure 5.41) and then return to the beginning position.

▼ **Leg Extension:** This machine isolates the quadriceps and takes them through a full range of motion, providing an intense second exercise for this muscle group. Use caution by starting the knee extension with the knee at no less than a 90-degree angle. This exercise improves walking, balance, rising from sitting to standing, and lowering from standing to sitting. Adjust the back of the seat so the centers of the knees align with the machine's pivot point. The leg pad should rest slightly above the ankles. The participant extends the legs fully and smoothly through the pain-free range of motion (figure 5.42) and then returns to the beginning position.

▼ **Lat Pull-Down:** This machine exercises the body's second-largest muscle group (the back), provides a second exercise for the biceps, and engages muscles important in stabilizing the shoulder joint. This exercise contributes to reaching, lifting, and carrying. Adjust the seat so the handgrips are just at the extended reach. Have the participant pull down to shoulder level (figure 5.43) and return to the extended position. Remind participants to pull the scapulas down and together on each repetition.

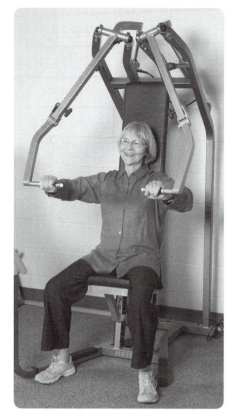

▶ **Figure 5.41** Seated chest press.

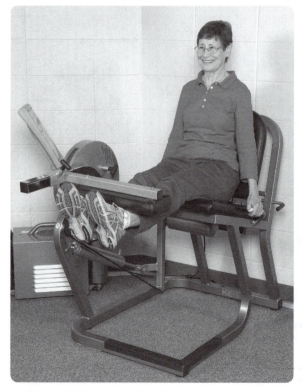

▶ **Figure 5.42** Leg extension.

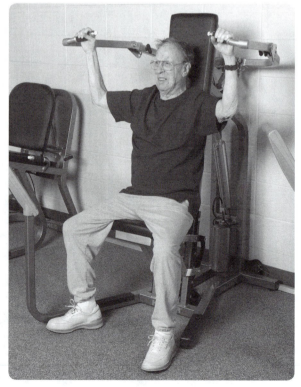

▶ **Figure 5.43** Lat pull-down.

▶ **Leg Curl:** This machine isolates the hamstrings, providing an intense second exercise for this muscle group. This exercise contributes to walking, balance, rising, and sitting. Adjust the back of the seat so the knees align with the machine's pivot point. The leg cushion should rest slightly above the heel, and the thigh cushion should fit snugly. Participants flex the knees through their full pain-free range of motion (figure 5.44) and then smoothly return to the beginning position.

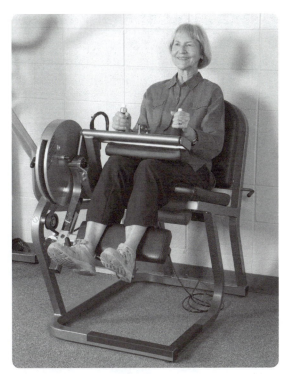

This six machine circuit provides a solid program to improve strength and power. If you have access to additional machines, the shoulder press and triceps press are good choices. The shoulder press exercise can improve the ability to lift objects overhead (household chores, traveling), and the triceps press exercise strengthens the muscles that assist in rising from a chair when leg strength is compromised.

▶ **Figure 5.44**   Leg curl.

■ **Shoulder (Military) Press:** This is another beneficial machine in that it isolates the deltoid muscles, which play an important role in stabilizing the shoulder joint. This exercise contributes to carrying and any overhead activity such as lifting something onto or off of a shelf. Adjust seat so the handgrips are just below shoulder level. Have the participant extend the arms overhead and then return to the beginning position.

■ **Triceps Press:** This machine isolates the triceps muscles, which are often used for assistance in rising from a chair. This exercise contributes to lifting, carrying, rising, and sitting. Adjust seat so the elbows are at close to full flexion. Have the participant press the hands down to extend the elbows fully.

If participants in your program don't have access to resistance training machines, they can start with ankle weights, handheld weights, and resistance bands. Be sure to choose props and equipment that allow for progressive resistance. When using ankle weights, participants should be able to increase the weight as they get stronger. Handheld weights should be in a variety of weights (from 1 pound to at least 5 pounds). Bands should be of at least three levels of resistance, and participants can use two bands (e.g., light and medium) together to increase the resistance.

For the best results, however, acquiring strength machines should be a high priority, even if your facility has to buy only one machine per year until you have a circuit to work with. Here is the recommended order for purchasing machines: leg press, chest press, upper back, leg extension, leg curl, and lat pull-down. The leg press machine works the entire lower body, and the chest press and upper back machines work most of the upper body. Even these three machines will foster significant gains in strength and power.

Consider looking for grant funds or mounting fund-raising campaigns for this important aspect of your fitness program. Visit www.keiser.com for a free downloadable resource that guides you through the process of finding and applying for grants focused on improving wellness in older adults.

▶ Training Strength and Power With Body Weight

Training strength with body weight requires that the muscles be challenged beyond what is normal for everyday activities. The key to training with body weight is to increase the difficulty of performing the exercise. For example, very sedentary people can improve leg strength by performing 8 to 10 leg extensions and then holding the leg in extension for 8 to 10 counts. Others can stand up and sit down 8 to 10 times to improve leg strength. Still others may improve strength by stepping up onto a stair and back down. In addition, doing push-ups against the wall or on the floor can improve upper-body strength.

To improve power with body weight, you must add the speed component. Coach clients to consciously *choose* to move as quickly as possible. It may have been a long time since they thought about moving quickly. Remember to weigh potential benefits against potential risks when creating programs. Always start by improving strength first and then add the speed component later. Make sure clients have balance support so they can concentrate on speed of movement rather than balance and speed.

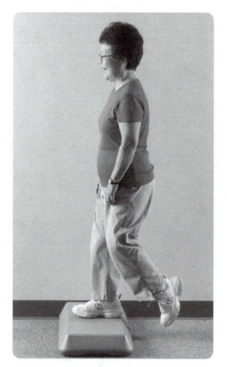

▶ **Figure 5.45** Step exercise.

Step Box

Use a sturdy box next to a wall or railing for balance support. Make sure it has a nonskid surface on both the bottom and the top. The lowest step in a flight of stairs can be used if a railing is available. Do not progress to a height greater than required for normal activities (e.g., climbing stairs, stepping onto a curb, or climbing into a bus or airplane). Maintaining good posture, participants should step fully onto and off of the box with each repetition, using balance support if necessary. Have clients practice balance separately so they can concentrate on speed.

1. **Step On and Off**
    a. Step onto and off of the step (figure 5.45), leading with the right foot. Step up (right), up (left), down (right), down (left); repeat 2 times.
    b. Repeat, leading with the left foot.
    c. To address power, repeat the full sequence by stepping up as quickly as possible while retaining good form. Step down under control at a lower speed.

2. **Step-Up With Knee Lift**
    a. Step onto the box with the right foot; swing left knee up to 90 degrees (figure 5.46).
    b. Bring left leg back down to the ground; repeat 4 times stepping up with right foot.
    c. Repeat 4 times stepping up with the left foot.
    d. For a more difficult progression, rise onto the toes when swinging the knee up to 90 degrees.
    e. To address power, repeat the sequence lifting the knee to 90 degrees as quickly as possible each time.

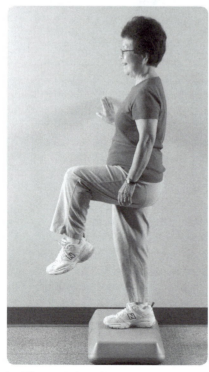

▶ **Figure 5.46** Step-up with knee lift.

Foot Power

These exercises develop the ability to respond to a trip or slip with quick foot movement. Please practice them with wall, railing, chair, or even walker support.

1. **Squash the Bugs (for foot speed)**

   a. Stamp as quickly as possible in all directions as if squashing ants around your feet (figure 5.47).

   b. Emphasize foot and leg speed, returning to center between each stamp. Be sure to stamp front, sideways, and behind, first using one foot and then the other.

   c. Now stomp (transfer weight), alternating right and left feet while squashing bugs as quickly as possible. This is like stomping the snow off of boots, but faster and in all directions!

2. **Power Steps**

   a. Face a wall, with hands ready to catch the wall if necessary.

   b. Starting with feet together, lean forward (with no bending at the hips). At the last moment take a quick step forward to avoid falling (figure 5.48). Repeat several times, "catching" with the right foot and then again with the left foot. Concentrate on delaying foot movement and recovering with speed.

   c. Repeat to the side if appropriate (requires more strength and balance). Lean sideways to the wall (without bending at the waist) and step sideways to avoid falling. This is an advanced move because it involves leaning onto the leg that has to be picked up to catch the fall. Repeat to the opposite side.

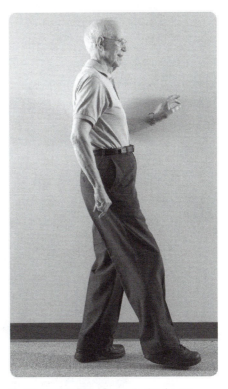

▶ **Figure 5.47** Squash the bugs.

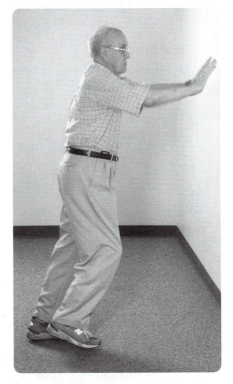

▶ **Figure 5.48** Power steps.

Arm Power

These exercises help develop arm speed so the arms can react to a near fall or catch body weight if a fall occurs. Participants work with a partner or against a wall. Use a large exercise ball, a lightweight medicine ball, a spongy ball, or a slightly deflated basketball. If balance is compromised, have the participant perform with support (e.g., with back to a wall or seated) and take care when bending over to retrieve a ball.

1. **Chest Pass**
   a. Perform a chest pass to a partner, as quickly as possible (figure 5.49).
   b. Concentrate on speed of elbow extension and shoulder flexion. Repeat 8 times.

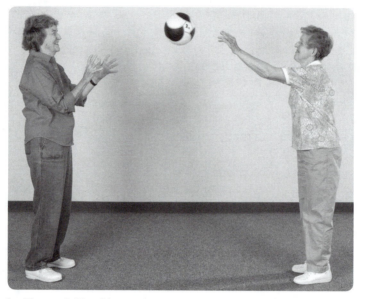

▶ **Figure 5.49** Chest pass.

2. **Floor Pass**
   a. Pass the ball to a partner by bouncing it forcefully so the rebound is high (figure 5.50).
   b. Concentrate on speed of movement. Repeat 8 times.

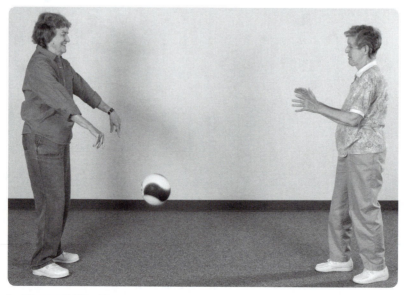

▶ **Figure 5.50** Floor pass.

The previous exercises for strength and power using body weight were adapted from a presentation at the 2004 World Congress on Physical Activity and Aging in London, Ontario, by Pommy Macfarlane. Using these exercises as examples, consider all of the activities that can be adapted to incorporate speed of movement. Always provide balance support when practicing speed of movement, and weigh the potential benefits against the potential risks for each activity.

WELLNESS WRAP-UP

A high-quality exercise program uses proper exercise techniques along with strategies that enhance other wellness dimensions, such as social connections and emotional well-being. Exercises must focus on movement that matters for your target group. This could mean chair exercises to help participants perform activities of daily living or vigorous exercises to facilitate competition in sports and activities that require aerobic endurance, agility, strength, and speed. Identify what you want to accomplish with each exercise session and match techniques to those goals.

Use the concept of wellness stations to provide opportunities for your clients to participate in wellness activities on their own. Integrate a function-based exercise with artwork and statements that promote self-responsibility and a positive approach to life.

Make the time in your program to address strength and power. They are both critical to retaining functional independence and quality of life. Lobby for resistance training equipment that allows you to safely train strength and power. Incorporate strength and power training activities using body weight into chair-exercise classes, low-impact aerobics, and even walking programs.

Water-Based Programming

ater-exercise programs enjoy wide appeal. Many physicians refer adults to water exercise to aid recovery from hip, knee, or back injury, and adults with balance or joint problems can safely perform vigorous exercise in the water. Water exercise has advantages over land-based exercise, such as providing resistance through the full range of motion and allowing participants to perform dynamic movement without creating impact on the joints. Many healthy, active clients enjoy the water and the vigorous but gentle workout it can provide.

This chapter discusses special concerns for water-exercise classes, including target heart rate variation in the water, water temperature, instructor requirements, pool safety, and appropriate music choices. The chapter provides specific programming for beginning water aerobics (level 1) and more vigorous water aerobics (level 2) and outlines specific modifications for arthritis water exercise. A large portion of the chapter describes and illustrates specific water exercises to use during warm-up, aerobic conditioning, cool-down, and stretching segments, including many flotation exercises. The aerobic exercises are arranged in groups from easiest to most strenuous:

- Transition exercises (very easy)
- Group 1 (low-intensity aerobics)
- Group 2 (moderate-intensity aerobics)
- Group 3 (high-intensity aerobics)
- Sample classes are provided that illustrate how to alternate between transition exercises and exercises from groups 1 to 3 to create the level appropriate for your group.

SPECIAL CONSIDERATIONS FOR WATER-EXERCISE CLASSES

Water exercise for adults carries special considerations. These considerations include knowing target heart rate variations appropriate to water exercise, teaching participants how to use the rating of perceived exertion, accounting for safety aspects unique to a pool environment, and maintaining a water temperature that allows for both comfort and safety of your participants. Music choices are also unique because of the generally poor acoustics in a pool area and the possibility that some participants will have uncorrected hearing impairments.

Target Heart Rate

Target heart rate zones for water exercise are different than those for land exercise. Many factors influence heart rates in the water. The Institute for Aerobic Research notes that horizontal exercise in the water (like lap swimming) brings about a heart rate 17 beats per minute lower than that achieved during land-based exercise, whereas a downward adjustment of 8 to 10 beats per minute applies to vertical exercise in the water (Pappas-Gaines, 1993). In addition, heart rates of clients exercising in a cool pool (78-83 degrees Fahrenheit, or 25-28 degrees Celsius) are approximately 15% lower than experienced on land, whereas warm water (84-88 degrees Fahrenheit, or 29-31 degrees Celsius) results in heart rates that are generally 10% lower than experienced on land. Depth of water also has an impact, with heart rates 8 to 11 beats per minute lower in chest-deep water than in waist-deep water (Sova, 2005).

Because of these variations and the influence of other factors such as air temperature and pool area ventilation, it is best to rely primarily on the rating of perceived exertion (explained in chapter 4 on page 59). However, I still recommend monitoring participants' heart rates along with their RPEs. Heart rates can offer important comparisons or benchmarks to call attention to a potential problem. For example, if a participant usually has a 10-second count of 17 beats and during class exhibits a count of 21, that change should draw your attention to monitor her more closely. See figure 6.1 for the Karvonen formula modified for adult water-exercise class, using the factor of 17 beats per minutes. Again, rely heavily on RPE but consider monitoring exercise heart rates as well for an extra measure of safety.

Train students to call out their RPE whenever you point to them while checking exercise intensity during class. Check exercise heart rates twice during aerobics, and have students call out their 10-second exercise pulse rates when you point to them during the heart rate check. When you ask participants to judge their levels of exertion or take their pulse rate, use the same clear, easy-to-follow commands each time, being sensitive to the fact that many participants who require vision or hearing correction will not be wearing their glasses or hearing aids while in the water.

Safety

The special conditions imposed by a pool environment present some additional safety concerns for

Resting heart rate (RHR)   To obtain an accurate RHR, count the pulse for 1 full minute after having been at complete rest for a minimum of 20 minutes.

Target heart rate (THR) zone   The average asymptomatic senior should be able to safely work between 50% and 75% of maximum HR during the aerobic phase.

10-second count   The pulse rate counted for 10 seconds is used as a quick check of heart rate during the aerobic phase.

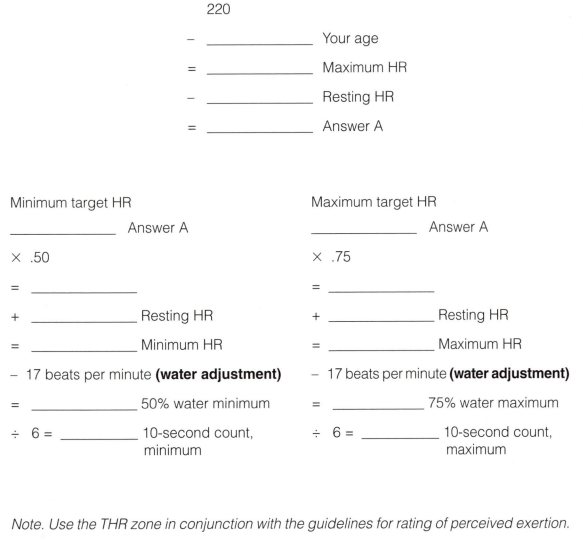

Land-based exercise training zone for seniors

220

− _____ Your age

= _____ Maximum HR

− _____ Resting HR

= _____ Answer A

Minimum target HR

_____ Answer A

× .50

= _____

+ _____ Resting HR

= _____ Minimum HR

− 17 beats per minute **(water adjustment)**

= _____ 50% water minimum

÷ 6 = _____ 10-second count, minimum

Maximum target HR

_____ Answer A

× .75

= _____

+ _____ Resting HR

= _____ Maximum HR

− 17 beats per minute **(water adjustment)**

= _____ 75% water maximum

÷ 6 = _____ 10-second count, maximum

Note. Use the THR zone in conjunction with the guidelines for rating of perceived exertion.

▶ **Figure 6.1**   Modified Karvonen formula for water exercise.

water-exercise programs. For example, in addition to having the CPR and first aid qualifications required of an exercise instructor for adults, a water-exercise instructor may need to have training in emergency water safety. If there is a lifeguard on duty during the water-exercise class, you may not be required to have emergency water safety training. However, if you alone will be responsible for the complete safety of the participants in the pool area, you must have lifeguard certification.

Poolside Versus In-Pool Teaching

When you have the responsibility of lifeguard as well as teacher, you must teach while standing on the pool deck. It is impossible to effectively monitor both the exercise participants and the entire pool area while in the water. Several other factors make it more advantageous for the instructor to teach on the poolside rather than in the pool.

First, participants with diminished levels of vision and hearing will find it very difficult to hear and see an instructor who is teaching from the water. Second, it is much easier for all class members to follow exercises that are being clearly demonstrated on the deck. Third, and most important, when teaching from the deck, you can clearly see each of the participants. This allows you to observe whether someone is performing an exercise incorrectly. It also provides you with continuous feedback from facial expressions, which means you are more

aware if someone is having difficulty with exercise intensity. Continuously monitoring each person's response to exercise is critical to maintaining the safety of an adult exercise class.

Pool Area

As a water-exercise instructor, you must consider the safety of your class participants from the moment they step into the pool area until they leave the facility. Evaluate the shower areas and pool deck for hazards such as slick spots or obstacles. If the shower or deck is slick, ask students to wear aqua shoes or some other type of nonskid shoe. Monitor the condition of ladders and stairs into the pool, and take the appropriate measures to remedy the situation if they become slick or unstable. Monitor the condition of the bottom of the pool to ensure that it is free of debris and does not pose any safety hazards.

Safe Movement

Exercising in the water provides a low-impact workout, but you must still take care to prevent injury to participants. To promote an injury-free class, avoid exercises that require rapid twisting and excessive jumping. Alternate the higher-impact jumping movements with movements that keep one foot on the pool bottom. Avoid jerky, out-of-the-water arm movements, which could cause or aggravate shoulder soreness. Avoid performing an excessive

Staying Healthy Together

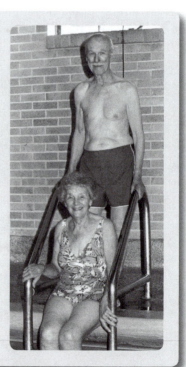

At the time of this photograph, Bill and Mary Walters had been taking the senior water-exercise class 2 or 3 times a week for 9 years. Asked what motivates them to keep coming on a regular basis, Mary replies, "It starts the day out right for me. I really miss it if we are gone."

"It makes me feel much better physically and mentally," Bill adds. Mary agrees and adds that it gives her a better outlook on life. "I'm glad Bill and I are committed to exercising together." Both Bill and Mary agree that water-exercise class helps them stay healthy together—a high priority for them.

amount of "hanging" wall exercises that require students to support their body weight with their hands, arms, and shoulders.

As you would with a land-based exercise program, weigh the potential risks against the benefits for each movement. Ask participants which exercises they enjoy doing and which exercises are uncomfortable to perform. Ask whether they believe they are achieving the desired results and whether they are experiencing any soreness after exercise. Continuous feedback from participants is essential to tailoring the class to meet their needs.

Pool Temperature

The temperature of the pool can have a significant impact on the success of a water-exercise program. If the water temperature is below 85 degrees Fahrenheit (29 degrees Celsius), it will likely be uncomfortable for participants who have arthritis or muscle and joint dysfunction. The Arthritis Foundation requires a minimum water temperature of 83 degrees Fahrenheit (28 degrees Celsius) to conduct its YMCA Arthritis Aquatics Program but recommends a temperature of 84 to 88 degrees Fahrenheit (29-31 degrees Celsius) (Sanders, 2008). A good pool temperature for adult water-exercise classes is 86 to 88 degrees Fahrenheit (30-31 degrees Celsius). This temperature allows for comfort during the warm-up and cool-down phases but is not so warm that it might pose a safety hazard during the aerobic phase. If water temperature is 90 degrees Fahrenheit (32 degrees Celsius) or above, do not attempt to do aerobic conditioning.

Finding a pool that offers a comfortable temperature is a challenge, because many pools cater to lap swimmers, who prefer a temperature ranging from 82 to 85 degrees Fahrenheit (27-29 degrees Celsius). If the only available pool is close to 82 degrees Fahrenheit (27 degrees Celsius), you will probably be unable to develop a successful water-exercise program for older adults. If the water temperature is closer to 85 degrees Fahrenheit (29 degrees Celsius), you may be able to adjust the structure of the class to work better at that temperature. For example, you can program more vigorous warm-up exercises to raise body temperature, such as water-walking forward, sideways, and backward; flutter kicks on the side of the pool or with jugs; and bicycling with jugs. You can use bicycling with jugs during strength work to keep the body temperature elevated during that phase.

After the aerobic phase, you can either shorten the cool-down and stretching phase or conduct the stretching session on the deck of the pool (not optimal). If you choose to leave the pool for the stretch session, be sure the air temperature is warm and the pool deck is safe. (Stretches can be done against the wall; see chapter 5 for descriptions and illustrations of wall exercises.) Before participants exit the pool to stretch, take time for them to reduce their heart rates by walking forward, backward, and sideways in the water. Exiting the pool without this cool-down can increase the risk of a rapid drop in blood pressure as a result of the difference between water and air pressure. Shortening the cool-down and stretching phase, or getting out of the pool for stretching, is definitely a compromise, but trying to stretch and relax in cold water can cause a rapid drop in body temperature and create excessive discomfort for participants.

Music

Music plays an essential role in participants' enjoyment of the class. Be aware of the poor acoustics that exist in most pool areas, and make the necessary adjustments in the volume and variety of music. The guidelines in chapter 4 on choosing music also apply to water exercise. The best choices for water exercise are simple, clear instrumentals with a strong, easy-to-follow beat. Simple vocals can also be used, but poor acoustics and splashing water will compete with the music and its vocal accompaniment. If you use vocals, alternate them with instrumental arrangements to provide a soothing balance of music.

GENERAL FORMAT

Water-exercise classes begin with a warm-up that involves gentle range of motion activities designed to promote circulation and help the participants become comfortable with movement. The warm-up should also offer opportunities for participants to interact with each other in the water and to interact with the instructor. Just as in land-based classes, you should facilitate social interaction and a sense of belonging. Classes include an aerobic phase that lasts from 15 to 25 minutes, depending on the participants' level of ability. These phases must include careful monitoring of exercise intensity; instruct participants to check their ratings of perceived exertion and pulse rates after the warm-up exercises and again at least twice during the aerobic phase. Immediately after the conclusion of the aerobic phase, ask participants to take their exercise pulse and determine their RPE. One minute later, have them determine their recovery pulse rate and RPE. Use the target heart rate variation described in figure 6.1, and remember that target heart rates in the water are affected by many factors, so they are most useful as a comparison that can alert you to a participant who may be having an unusual response to exercise that day. (Specific strategies for monitoring exercise intensity are presented in chapter 4.)

Include coordination movements in the warm-up and aerobic phases, varying arm movements with opposition, same-side (unison), and sequential motions. This will keep the class interesting while participants develop and improve coordination skills. Remind participants to touch their heels to the pool floor frequently so they do not stay on the balls of their feet throughout the class. Keeping all body weight on the balls of the feet throughout the class period can seriously overwork the gastrocnemius (calf) muscle, causing soreness and possible injury.

A cool-down and stretching phase follows the aerobics and should involve all major muscle groups. Water-walking for several minutes is a good way to make sure everyone's heart rate returns to an acceptable level. Pay close attention to stretching the gastrocnemius muscles, the low back, and the hamstrings, which will have been worked repeatedly during the aerobic phase. Use both the pool wall and the center of the pool for stretching exercises. Use slow, gentle stretches with no sharp movements, and develop smooth stretching sequences that promote relaxation as well as flexibility.

Level 1 Class Format

A level 1 class is appropriate for clients who want a full-body workout but have low aerobic capacity or musculoskeletal issues. Clients in a level 1 class may be uncomfortable in the water or may simply prefer a more gentle exercise session. Each class consists of approximately 20 to 25 minutes of warm-up, range of motion, and strength work. It should also have 15 to 20 minutes of aerobics and 20 to 25 minutes of cool-down, stretching, and relaxation work. Use transition movements such as jogging and sculling side to side between high- and medium-intensity aerobic movements. Spend an equal amount of time in the transition movements as in the higher-intensity movements. For example, have participants perform 16 to 24 knee lifts (medium intensity), jog in place for 16 to 24 counts (transition), perform 16 to 24 cross-country skiers (high intensity), and then

scull side to side for 16 to 24 counts (transition). As participants become more fit, have them perform a higher number of the medium- or high-intensity movements (e.g., 24), followed by a lower number of the transition movements (e.g., 16). Another approach is to spend 30 to 40 seconds doing a medium- or high-intensity movement followed by 30 to 40 seconds of a transition movement. As the participants become more physically fit, have them perform the transition movements for a shorter duration (e.g., 30 seconds) than the medium- or high-intensity movements (e.g., 40 seconds).

Level 2 Class Format

A level 2 water aerobics class is appropriate for clients who want a more intense aerobic workout. It consists of approximately 15 to 20 minutes of warm-up, range of motion, and strength work. It also includes 20 to 25 minutes of aerobics and 15 to 20 minutes of cool-down, stretch, and relaxation movements. You may use transition movements between medium- and high-intensity exercises, but spend more time in the high- and medium-intensity aerobic movements. For example, have participants do 24 to 32 knee lifts (medium intensity), jog in place for 16 to 20 counts (transition), perform 24 to 32 cross-country skiers (high intensity), and then scull side to side for 16 to 20 counts (transition). In the level 2 class, you can use low- and medium-intensity exercises consecutively without a transition exercise. For example, have exercisers do 16 to 24 knee lifts (medium intensity), perform 16 to 24 large kicks front (medium intensity), and then jog in place 16 to 20 counts (transition). An even higher level of aerobic conditioning can be gained by performing two high-intensity exercises consecutively without a transition movement between them; as always, carefully weigh the benefits against the potential risks.

Using the time approach, have level 2 participants spend 40 to 50 seconds doing a medium- or high-intensity exercise followed by 15 to 20 seconds of a transition exercise. As participants become more physically fit, have them perform the medium- and high-intensity exercises consecutively without a transition exercise. When performing consecutive exercises, limit the combined time spent in low- and medium-intensity movements to approximately 80 seconds before returning to a transition exercise. For example, spend 30 to 40 seconds doing knee lifts (medium intensity) and 30 to 40 seconds doing large kicks (medium intensity), followed by 20 seconds doing a transition exercise. See the sidebar for a sample water-exercise class.

SAMPLE WATER-EXERCISE CLASS (LEVEL 1)

Music: See chapter 4, page 50. Start with warm-up music; the faster-tempo aerobics songs like Glen Miller's "Chattanooga Choo-Choo" work the best.

5 Minutes of Water-Walking

Walk forward, backward, and sideways across the shallow end of the pool. Start with no music, because this is a good time to visit with participants and encourage interaction.

10 Minutes of Range of Motion Exercises

Neck range of motion exercises alternating with shoulder shrugs and circles

Arm swings: front to back, then opening side and crossing front

Small circles performed with the whole arm

Torso isolations to the front and back, side to side, and circles

Hip movements side to side and then in circles clockwise and counterclockwise

One-leg swings

Ankle circles

Knee extensions

Flutter kicks on the wall

Sunrise, sunset

Instruct participants to grab flotation devices for strength work.

10 Minutes of Flotation Work

Bicycling (arms tucked)

Mermaid side to side (arms extended)

Bicycling (arms tucked)

Pinwheel (arms extended or tucked)

Mermaid front to back (arms extended)

Bicycling (arms tucked)

Scissors (arms extended)

Pinwheel (arms extended or tucked)

Bicycling (arms tucked)

Mermaid side to side (arms extended)

Mermaid front to back (arms extended)

Bicycling (arms tucked)

Instruct participants to place flotation devices on pool deck and check pulses and ratings of perceived exertion.

15 Minutes of Aerobic Exercises

Sequence A

Jogging in place for 20 seconds

Rocking horse, 15 seconds right leg front, 15 seconds left leg front

Sculling side to side 20 seconds

Small kicks front 20 seconds, arms swinging in opposition

(continued)

Jogging in place 20 seconds, arms pressed out front and in, then side and in

Rocking horse side to side for 30 seconds

Knee lifts front 20 seconds

Sculling side to side 20 seconds

Repeat sequence A, and then check pulses and ratings of perceived exertion.

Sequence B

Knee lifts front 15 seconds, cross-knee lift 15 seconds; repeat

Jogging in place 20 seconds

Large kicks to the front, arms reaching forward in opposition 20 seconds

Sculling side to side 20 seconds

Karate kicks side to side 20 seconds

Sculling side to side 20 seconds

Jogging forward 8 counts, 4 jumping jacks, jogging back 8 counts, 4 jumping jacks (20 seconds)

Sculling side to side 20 seconds

Side knee lifts with elbows to knees 15 seconds, cross-knee lifts 15 seconds

Jogging in place 20 seconds

Frog jumps for 20 seconds

Sculling side to side 16 counts, 4 cross-country skiers, repeating for a total of 30 seconds

Repeat sequence B for a total of 15 minutes of aerobic conditioning.

Check pulses immediately and assess ratings of perceived exertion.

Cool-Down and Stretch

Water-walk forward, backward, and sideways 1 minute (check pulses and exertion again for indication of recovery).

Continue water-walking in various patterns for 5 minutes.

Wall stretches

Rock-back

Achilles stretch

Cross knee

Hamstring stretch

Quad stretch

Center pool stretches

Ear to shoulder

Cross arm

Balance activities

Hand and finger mobility

Contraction

Hug and stretch

Deep breathing

Grab flotation devices and float in water with quiet music.

For a level 2 class. gradually increase the time spent doing medium- to high-intensity exercises. Decrease the time spent in transition exercises but maintain at least 10 seconds for each transition exercise.

▶ Specific Water Exercises

The following specific exercises can be used in both the level 1 and level 2 water-exercise classes. The warm-up can be very similar for both levels, but for the level 1 class, program fewer repetitions of strength, wall, and flotation exercises (e.g., exercises performed with water bells, noodles, or empty gallon milk jugs for flotation).

Match the aerobic level to the class level by striking a balance between the transition movements and the higher-intensity aerobic movements. The warm-up and cool-down phases also provide a time for socializing, giving health tips, and sharing bits of wisdom or humor. If the water temperature is comfortable, devote a few minutes at the end of class to total relaxation, allowing participants to float in the water and relax with the lights turned down and quiet music to create a pleasant atmosphere.

Warm-Up

In addition to including warm-up exercises, this phase includes range of motion and strength exercises, all of which are designed to promote circulation and prepare the body for more vigorous movement. Start working from the head down, and move each joint through the range of motion you will use during the aerobic phase of the program. Do not attempt to increase flexibility during this phase, but only move through the comfortable range of motion for each muscle and joint. Part of the warm-up can include flotation work or strength and range of motion. Water bells or noodles are preferred equipment because the small handles of milk jugs can be difficult to hold or may cause discomfort for those with arthritis. However, in the absence of a budget for equipment, gallon milk jugs or large-handled laundry detergent jugs work well as flotation devices. Remind participants to be conscious of whether exercise with jugs aggravates arthritis symptoms, and make alternatives available.

Center Pool Warm-Ups

- **Water-Walking:** Have students walk back and forth across the pool, using long strides and emphasizing the proper foot-strike pattern of heel and then ball of the foot (no flat-footed steps). Water-walking can also be done moving either backward (with a foot strike of toe–ball–heel) or sideways (stepping directly to the side). For variety, have students walk forward or backward or walk sideways while crossing the right foot in front of the left and then the left foot in front of the right. Water-walking offers a great opportunity for social interaction. Have students walk toward and away from each other or move in a large circle, and have lines cross over each other or weave in and out. Partner work is also fun. Give students a task, for example, finding out what their partner had for breakfast that morning, to encourage connections.
- **Power Water-Walking:** Have exercisers walk back and forth across the pool with knees bent, taking small steps. This can be done forward, backward, or sideways or crossing the right foot in front of the left and then the left foot in front of the right.
- **Small Prances:** Using a foot placement of toe–ball–heel to articulate the foot and ankle, exercisers prance in place or while moving across the pool.
- **Bicycling:** Participants bicycle forward or backward with flotation devices tucked under the arms to warm up the entire lower body.
- **Flutter Kicks:** With kickboards or flotation devices held out in front of the body, participants do flutter kicks while moving across the pool.
- **Neck Range of Motion Exercise:** Any of the neck exercises outlined in chapter 5 can be used in a water-exercise warm-up. Choose two or three to begin your class. Alternate neck exercises with shoulder exercises to avoid fatiguing the neck muscles.

- **Shoulder Movement:** Any of the shoulder exercises outlined in chapter 5 can be used in a water-exercise warm-up. Choose two or three exercises for this phase of your class. For variety, add knee bends to shoulder exercises (keep the feet flat on the pool bottom).
- **Arm Swings:** Participants swing one or both arms in unison or opposition forward and backward; they can also swing one or both arms across the front or back of the body.
- **Torso Movement:** The torso isolations, contraction, and rotation exercises described in chapter 5 work very well in the water-exercise warm-up. When performing contraction exercises, participants should bend both knees while contracting and then straighten the knees while opening the arms to the sides. When doing rotation exercises, participants should bend the knees during the rotation to the side and straighten when returning to neutral.
- **Hip Circles:** Exercisers begin by gently pushing their hips from side to side and then draw circles with their hips, clockwise and counterclockwise.
- **Toe-Drawing:** Pulling their toes along the pool floor, participants draw circles, squares, or any shape or write their names, addresses, and phone numbers using the foot only. For variation, participants may write much bigger by using the entire leg as the writing instrument, moving the knee and hip joints as well.
- **Single-Leg Swings:** With the weight on the left foot, exercisers swing the right leg forward and back (8 times) using the full range of motion at the hip while keeping the back straight and abdominals engaged; then they repeat the movement keeping the weight on the right foot and swinging the left leg. This exercise can also be done by opening and closing either leg to the side or crossing one leg in front or behind the other. (Flotation devices or the wall can be used for balance.)
- **Ankle Circles:** Exercisers bring the right knee to the chest and do right ankle circles (8 counts); then extend the leg (4 counts), hold (4 counts), and point and flex the foot for 8 to 16 counts (2 counts each); and then bend the knee back to the chest and repeat the sequence, beginning with the ankle circles. Then they switch to the opposite leg and begin by drawing the left knee to the chest.
- **Knee Extensions:** Participants bring the right knee to the chest (2 counts), extend the knee (2 counts), flex the knee (2 counts), and then repeat extensions and flexions for 8 to 12 counts. They repeat the exercise with the opposite leg.
- **Relevé:** Exercisers begin in neutral position and rise onto their toes (counts 1, 2), hold (3, 4, 5, 6), bend the knees (7, 8), hold (1, 2, 3, 4), bring the heels down flat on the pool floor (5, 6), and then straighten the legs (7, 8).
- **Balance Transfer:** Standing with the feet pointing straight forward and approximately 18 to 24 inches (45-60 centimeters) apart, participants rise onto their toes (counts 1, 2), transfer all of their weight to the right foot (3, 4), and flex the left knee and lift the left heel toward the buttock (5, 6, 7, 8); then they hold their balance (1, 2, 3, 4), return the left foot to the pool floor (5, 6), and return to beginning position. They repeat by transferring the weight to the left foot and lifting the right heel.

Warm-Ups at the Wall

Participants can do warm-ups with their right or left sides to the wall, facing the wall, or with their backs to the wall. Hanging from the wall can place undue stress on shoulder joints that may already be compromised by muscle weakness or joint dysfunction, so use wall-supported warm-ups where feet are off the pool floor (see photos *a-c*) sparingly and always with other warm-ups between wall-supported movements. Instruct participants to modify or avoid any exercises that cause discomfort and to exercise only through the pain-free range of motion.

▼ **Flutter Kicks:** Participants face the wall with the body floating on the surface of the water and do flutter kicks (figure 6.2a). Vary the size and tempo of the movement from small and fast to large and slow, remind participants to keep abdominal muscles engaged, and have the class kick a maximum of 1 minute at a time. This exercise can also be done with backs to the wall and arms in the pool gutter; participants flex at the hips until their legs are at a 90-degree angle (backs remain against the wall; figure 6.2b). An easier variation is to allow the body to come away from the wall and float on the surface of the water while doing the flutter kicks (figure 6.2c).

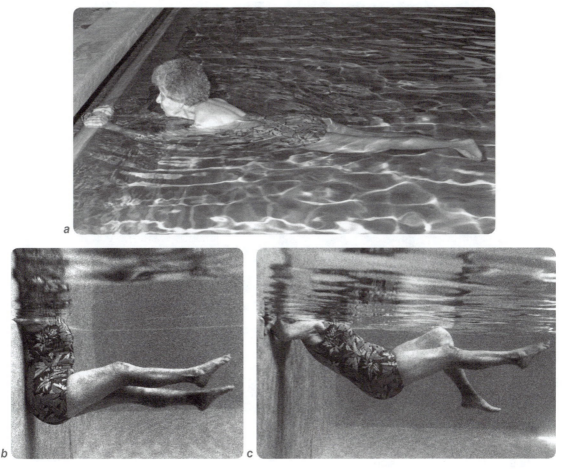

▶ **Figure 6.2** *(a)* Flutter kicks facing wall; *(b)* back to wall with legs at 90 degrees; *(c)* back to wall with legs out.

■ **Side Leg Lifts:** Exercisers stand with left sides to the wall, feet parallel, and lift the right leg directly to the side with some force (this creates more water resistance). Next they gently lower the leg back to neutral, repeating the entire movement 8 to 10 times. Then they switch to the opposite side.

■ **Side Leg Closes:** Participants do the side leg lift except they allow their legs to gently float open to the side and then apply force to close them back to neutral. They repeat the movement 8 to 10 times and then switch to the opposite side.

■ **Sunrise, Sunset:** Standing in right-side neutral position, exercisers lift the right knee to the right elbow, bending slightly at the waist to the right (counts 1, 2) and then return the right foot to the floor while extending the right arm over the head and bending slightly at the waist to the left (3, 4); they repeat the movement 8 to 10 times and then switch to the opposite side.

Flotation Exercises

Flotation exercise is generally done in water deep enough to allow the legs to move freely without touching the bottom of the pool. Special water-exercise equipment like water bells or noodles are ideal because they are easiest on the hands, but large plastic jugs (empty gallon milk jugs or laundry detergent) also work well as flotation aids. None of these props should be regarded as lifesaving devices, however, so those without swimming skills should stay in a pool depth at which they are comfortable for the flotation work.

Alternate flotation work that requires arms to be extended at shoulder level (figure 6.3) with those where the device is tucked under the arm (figure 6.6). Keeping the arms extended for the entire period of flotation work places unnecessary stress on the shoulder joints. Bicycling forward or backward with flotation devices tucked under the arms can be done between the exercises requiring arm extension. The neutral position is defined as having both legs hanging straight down. Most flotation exercises can be performed for 16 to 24 counts.

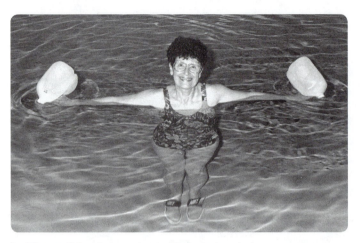

▶ **Figure 6.3** Jug work position—extended.

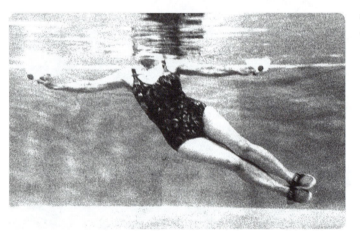

▶ **Figure 6.4** Mermaid side to side.

◀ **Mermaid Side to Side:** With arms extended to the sides and legs in neutral position, the exerciser brings the knees to the chest, pushes both legs straight out to the right, brings knees to chest again, and then pushes both legs straight out to the left (figure 6.4). The abdominal muscles are contracted each time the knees are brought to the chest.

◀ **Mermaid Front to Back:** This is like the mermaid side to side, except the legs are extended to the front and then to the back after the knees are brought to the chest (figure 6.5). Offer variation by having exercisers perform a mermaid front, side, back, and side.

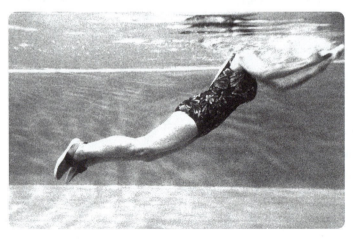

▶ **Figure 6.5** Mermaid front to back.

▼ **Pinwheel:** With the body at about a 45-degree angle and flotation devices either tucked under the arms (figure 6.6a) or extended to the side, the exerciser bicycles forward in a tight circle to the left (figure 6.6b), reverses the pinwheel by bicycling backward, and then switches to the opposite side and repeats.

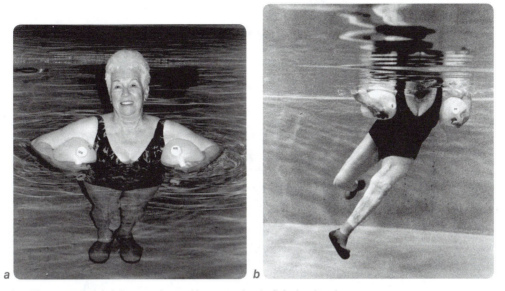

a   b

▶ **Figure 6.6** *(a)* Jug work position—tucked; *(b)* pinwheel.

▼ **Bell:** With flotation devices tucked under the arms or extended to the sides and legs in neutral position, the exerciser pulls the knees up and out to the sides and places the soles of the feet together (figure 6.7). Vary the exercise by having the exerciser swing the bent legs from side to side like the clapper in a bell.

▼ **Scissors:** With flotation devices tucked under the arms or extended to the sides and legs in neutral position, the exerciser opens the straight legs as far as possible (with the right going front and the left going back) (figure 6.8) and then switches so the left goes front and the right goes back. Introduce a variation using the arms in opposition to the legs.

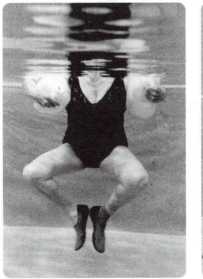

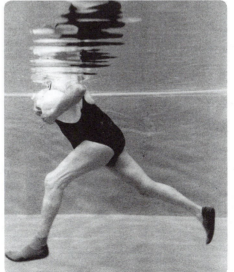

▶ **Figure 6.7** Bell.   ▶ **Figure 6.8** Scissors.

▼ **Pumps:** Beginning in neutral position with flotation devices extended to the sides (figure 6.9a), the exerciser pulls the knees to the chest, extends the legs out to the front (in a sitting position), flutter-kicks the legs to an open position, pumps the legs—right, left, right, left—by alternately flexing and extending the knees (figure 6.9b), flutter-kicks back to a sitting position, pulls the knees to the chest, and returns legs to neutral.

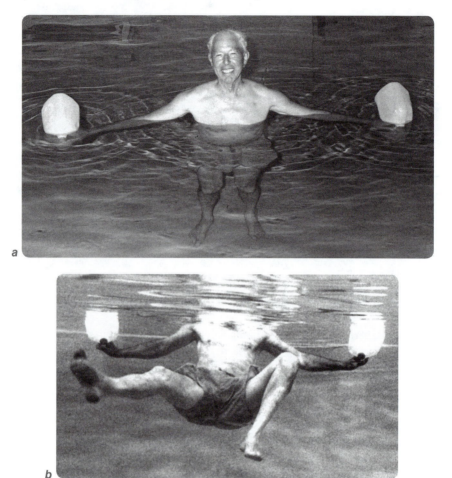

a

b

▶ **Figure 6.9** *(a)* Beginning position for pumps. *(b)* Pumps.

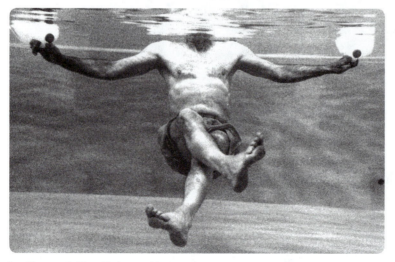

▶ **Figure 6.10** Sitting scissors.

◀ **Sitting Scissors:** Beginning in neutral position with flotation devices extended to the sides (see photo showing the beginning position for pumps), the exerciser does the motion sequence described in the pumps but instead of pumping with the legs while in the open sitting position, the participant pulls the legs closed, open, closed, open (figure 6.10); flutter-kicks back to the sitting position, and returns the legs to neutral.

- **Open and Close Side:** With flotation devices extended to the sides and legs in neutral position, the exerciser opens the straight legs as far as possible to the sides, then pulls the legs closed. You can vary this exercise by using force on the open, on the close, or on both open and close.
- **Abdominal Contraction:** Beginning in neutral position with flotation devices extended to the sides, the exerciser pulls the knees to the chest while contracting the abdominal muscles and then returns to neutral.
- **Hip Tuck:** Beginning in neutral, arms extended, the exerciser brings her knees to her chest, extends legs straight forward until lying on her back in the water, does a hip tuck by contracting the lower abdominals and tilting the pelvis under, holds the tuck 4 to 8 counts, and then releases.
- **Arm Flotation Work:** Arm flotation work is done in the shallow end of the pool in water approximately chest deep. The flotation devices, which are kept on the surface of the water, can be pushed forward and then pulled back to the chest, pushed out to the sides, or pushed front and opened to the sides. You can increase the resistance by having exercisers push the flotation devices slightly below the water surface while performing the exercises. The devices (either together or one at a time) can be pushed under the water toward the feet. When devices are pushed under the water, they should be kept close to the body rather than extended to the sides or front, which causes too much stress on the shoulder joints. Alternate exercises that keep the devices on the water surface with exercises that push the devices underwater. Because pushing devices under the water can exert a lot of pressure on the hands, do a maximum of 5 repetitions of underwater work. If the class is using empty plastic jugs, use only one jug and push it underwater using *both hands* on the body of the jug while pushing it toward the feet. Finally, remind participants to perform only exercises that are pain free.

Aerobics

I have divided the aerobic exercises into four groups: the transition group (low intensity, low impact), group 1 (low to medium intensity, low impact), group 2 (medium to high intensity, low impact), and group 3 (high intensity, higher impact). To provide another measure of safety to the aerobic phase, carefully alternate transition exercises with medium- and high-intensity exercises. Structuring your class this way allows participants to fit the intensity of the workout to their own needs.

Transition movements can be done with minimal effort by those who wish to bring their heart rates down or more vigorously by those who wish to maintain a higher level. Frequent use of transition movements also prevents overexposure to the higher-intensity jumping movements. Even in the water, these high-impact group 3 exercises, when used too frequently or too long, increase the potential for injury to participants with joint dysfunction.

Transition Exercises

Transition exercises consist of jogging in place and sculling side to side. Use these exercises to ease participants into the aerobics segment and then throughout the session to moderate the intensity of the workout.

- **Jogging in Place:** Exercisers jog lightly with small leg movement while keeping the arm work below shoulder level. Participants who want to keep their heart rates higher can jog more vigorously, lifting their knees higher and working harder with their arms.
- **Sculling Side to Side:** Participants do small kicks (approximately 6 inches [15 centimeters] wide) to diagonal right, left, right, left, while swaying both arms from side to side in unison with the legs. Participants who want to keep their heart rates high can kick higher and actively pull their arms through the water.

Group 1 Exercises

Group 1 exercises are low- to medium-intensity, low-impact movements. They are good exercises for beginning the aerobics phase and to use alternately with group 2 exercises later in the session.

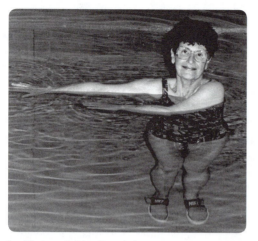

▶ **Figure 6.11**   Pendulum.

◀ **Pendulum:** Begin with both arms to the right and parallel to the floor. Pull arms through the water like a pendulum moving to the left parallel position (figure 6.11). Exercisers can perform this movement standing or can step from side to side in unison with arm motion.

▼ **Rocking Horse Front:** Exercisers rock forward on the right foot and backward on the left, using their arms (held to the sides with elbows slightly flexed) to pull backward during the rock forward and forward during the rock backward (figure 6.12) then they switch sides, rocking forward on the left foot and backward on the right.

▼ **Rocking Horse Side:** Exercisers rock broadly to the right side on the right foot (right arm reaching to the right) and then to the left side on the left foot (left arm reaching to the left) (figure 6.13).

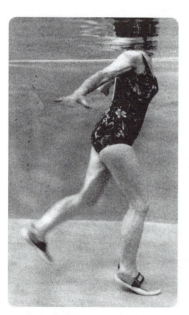

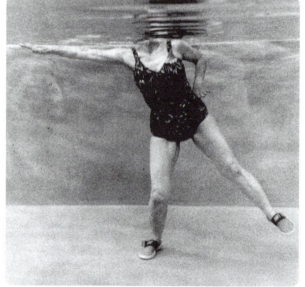

▶ **Figure 6.12**   Rocking horse front to back.

▶ **Figure 6.13**   Rocking horse side to side.

■ **Jogging Through the Water:** Participants jog forward or backward through the water, using the resistance of the water to increase the exercise intensity.

■ **Bicycling:** Bicycling with flotation devices can be done at low intensity for the warm-up (bicycling slowly) and at higher intensity for the aerobic phase (bicycling more vigorously).

Group 2 Exercises

Group 2 exercises are medium- to high-intensity exercises with low-impact movements, which effectively elevate the heart rate without any unnecessary jarring motions. Each of these exercises can be performed keeping one foot in contact with the pool floor (no jarring) or jumping from foot to foot (higher intensity with a small amount of jarring).

▼ **Knee Lifts:** Exercisers do knee lifts to the front with arms front (figure 6.14a). The class can also do knee lifts to the sides (figure 6.14b), right elbow touching the right knee, left elbow touching the left knee; or cross-knee lifts (figure 6.14c), left elbow touching the right knee, right elbow touching the left knee.

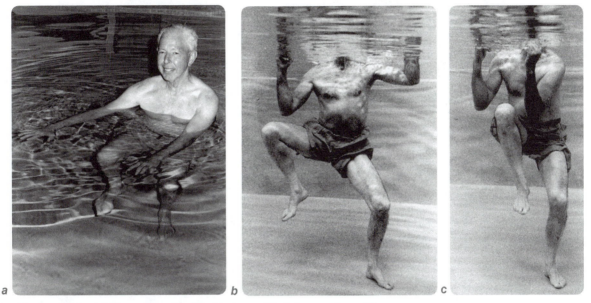

a   b   c

▶ **Figure 6.14** (a) Front knee lift; (b) side knee lift; (c) cross-knee lift.

▶ **Karate Kicks:** These are large kicks in which the right leg kicks out to the right side and then the left leg kicks to the left side (figure 6.15).

▪ **Front Kicks:** Exercisers do large kicks to the front with the arms pushing forward in opposition. Vary this exercise by having students reach for their shins or their toes on each kick.

▪ **Flutter Kicks:** Using flotation devices, exercisers flex at the hips and do flutter kicks to the front or, with the body straight and legs outstretched behind, flutter-kick across the pool. Participants also may do flutter kicks with their backs to the wall, arms in the pool gutter, or facing the wall and holding on to the pool gutter. For variety, alternate large, slow flutter kicks with small, fast flutter kicks. This exercise is most easily used at the beginning or end of the aerobic phase.

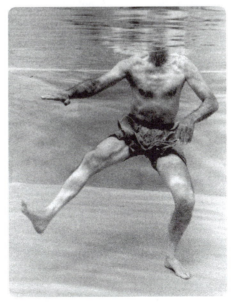

▶ **Figure 6.15** Karate kicks.

▼ **Flappers Front:** See figure 6.16 for upper-body position in all flapper movements. Exercisers lift the right foot to the front, touch it with the left hand (knee is turned out to the side) (figure 6.17), and return to neutral; next they lift the left foot to the front, touch it with the right hand, and return to neutral.

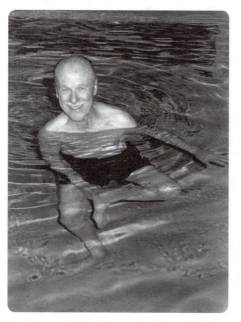

▶ **Figure 6.16** Upper-body position—flappers.

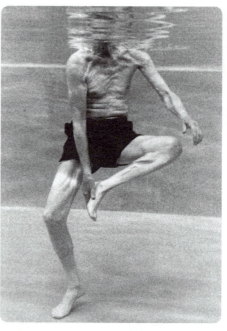

▶ **Figure 6.17** Flappers front.

▼ **Flappers Side:** Exercisers lift the right foot to the right side, touch it with the right hand (knee is turned in toward the center) (figure 6.18), and return to neutral; then they lift the left foot to the left side, touch it with the left hand, and return to neutral.

▼ **Flappers Back:** Exercisers lift the right foot back, cross it behind the left leg, touch the right foot with the left hand (figure 6.19), and return to neutral; they lift the left foot back, cross it behind the right leg, touch the left foot with the right hand, and return to neutral.

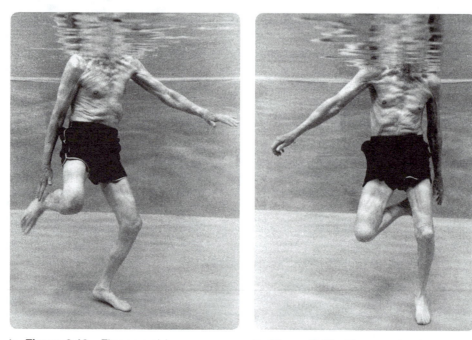

▶ **Figure 6.18** Flappers side.

▶ **Figure 6.19** Flappers back.

Group 3 Exercises

Group 3 includes high-intensity, higher-impact movements. The term *high-impact* is used comparatively rather than literally, because the water prevents all movements from being truly high impact. Use a transition exercise immediately before and after a group 3 exercise. Because you are teaching from the deck of the pool, you should not perform the high-impact exercises. Instead, demonstrate one or two of the exercises slowly so participants are clear on what they should do, and then do a low-impact version while on the deck. Try to match your exercise rhythm and speed with those in the pool. It may seem like you are demonstrating in slow motion, but remember that participants are performing the exercise against water resistance.

▼ **Cross-Country Skier:** Exercisers alternate jumping into a lunge position (left leg forward and right leg back, then right leg forward and left leg back) (figure 6.20a) while swinging the arms in opposition (figure 6.20b).

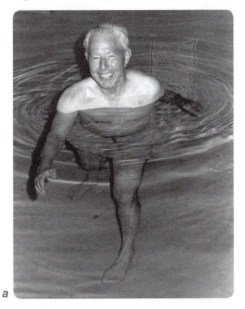

a

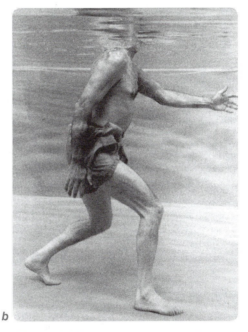

b

▶ **Figure 6.20** *(a)* Cross-country skier—upper body; *(b)* cross-country skier—lower body.

▶ **Cross Jump:** Exercisers jump up and land with the feet crossed and the arms crossed in front, then jump up and land with the feet and the arms open to the sides (figure 6.21).

▶ **Frog Jump:** Exercisers pull both feet up under the body at the same time with the knees pointing out to the sides (figure 6.22) and then return to a standing position.

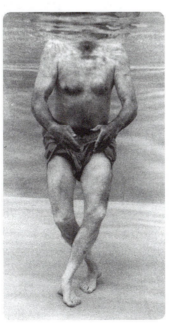

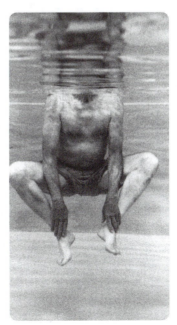

▶ **Figure 6.21** Cross jump.　▶ **Figure 6.22** Frog jump.

- **Jumping Jack:** Exercisers perform a standard jumping jack, arms opening to the sides as the legs open and closing next to the body as the legs come together. The class can also open their arms to the sides on the jump open and cross them in front on the jump together.
- **Tuck Jump:** Exercisers pull both feet up together while bringing their knees to the chest into a tuck position with arms wrapped around the knees; then they return to a standing position.
- **Jump:** With feet together, exercisers make small jumps forward and backward or side to side.
- **Double Knee Bounce:** Exercisers lift the right knee while hopping on the left foot, then jump with feet together, do another right knee lift while hopping on the left foot, and then jump with feet together. Repeat the movement lifting the left knee.
- **Traveling Movements:** Exercisers may also do jumping jacks, frog jumps, and tuck jumps while moving through the water, which makes them even higher-intensity exercises because of the increased resistance. Use traveling group 3 exercises sparingly and only in a level 2 class.

Cool-Down

The cool-down phase consists of slow, controlled movements that bring the heart rate down slowly and stretching exercises that help maintain or increase range of motion. Stretching exercises can be performed both in the center of the pool and at the pool wall. Relaxation movements are an excellent way to finish the class.

Center Pool

- **Water-Walking:** Exercisers walk slowly back and forth across the pool until the heart rate drops 4 to 5 beats below the exercise heart rate. Water-walking works very well as a transition between the aerobic phase and the cool-down and before taking the recovery heart rate.
- **Slow Bicycling:** Using flotation devices, exercisers bicycle slowly forward and backward.

Many of the warm-up movements that focus on range of motion can also be used in the cool-down phase (e.g., shoulder movements, arm swings, neck movements, torso contraction, balance work, and knee cross). During the cool-down phase, work to gently increase flexibility rather than simply pass through a range of motion. For interest and variety, exercisers can do some of the cool-down movements while standing in a circle. This promotes social interaction between students and is a good time to integrate other dimensions of well-being. For example, bring a thought for the day to share with students, find out what plans participants have for the rest of the week, or ask whether there is anything interesting going on in town. Consider dimming the lights during the last few minutes of the cool-down to allow participants to float, relax, and form their intentions for the rest of the day.

In the following exercises, neutral position is standing with the weight distributed evenly on both feet, arms hanging in a relaxed position to the sides.

- **Ear to Shoulder:** Exercisers gently drop right ear toward right shoulder and return to neutral, left ear toward left shoulder and return to neutral, and chin toward the chest and return to neutral. The shoulders must remain down and relaxed throughout the exercise. Use an 8- to 12-count hold in each position.
- **Cross Arm:** Exercisers reach the right arm across the front of the chest to the left, hold the right forearm with the left hand, and gently stretch the right shoulder (8-12 counts); then they release the right arm, open it to the right side, cross the right arm behind the back, grasp the right arm with the left hand and hold (8-12 counts), and release and return to neutral. They then repeat entire sequence with the left arm crossing the chest to the right.
- **Triceps Stretch:** Exercisers reach the right arm over the head and flex the elbow to touch the back (elbow pointing to ceiling), then reach across with the left hand and assist the triceps stretch by gently pulling the right elbow toward the left; they then release the arm, return to neutral, and repeat the movement on the opposite side.
- **Contraction:** Exercisers round their backs and press grasped hands forward while bending the knees. (Do not allow participants to sink down to round the back.) Then they straighten their backs while straightening the legs and opening the arms out to sides, and return to neutral.

- **Balance Activities:** Exercisers rise onto their toes, balance, transfer their weight from both feet to one foot only, balance, return to both feet, and then press heels down and bend the knees. To make the balance more difficult, add arm movements to the sides and over the head.
- **Hug and Stretch:** Exercisers wrap their arms across the front of the chest (hug) and drop the chin toward the chest, lift the chin to neutral while lifting the elbows up over the head and straightening the arms as if pulling a sweater off over the head, and return the arms to neutral.
- **Deep Breathing:** Exercisers take a deep breath in and rise onto their toes, opening their arms to the sides; then they exhale while pressing their heels back to the floor and bending their knees, with one arm crossing in front of the body and the other arm crossing in back.
- **Hand and Finger Mobility:** Hand and finger exercises can also be done in the water. For example, exercisers can alternately close the hand to a fist (as if grasping the water) and open the hand (as if throwing the water), do finger circles in the water (one finger at a time), pull open hands through the water, or form a circle with finger and thumb and flick the water. See chapter 5 for other wrist, hand, and finger exercises.

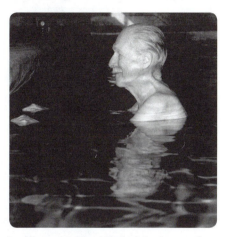

▶ **Figure 6.23** Neutral-facing wall position.

Wall Exercises

The positions used in wall stretches include neutral facing (figure 6.23), neutral back, right-side neutral, and left-side neutral.

- ▼ **Rock-Back:** Beginning in neutral-facing position with hands gripping the gutter, exercisers rock back on their heels while flexing their feet, hold (figure 6.24), return to neutral, then bring the chest to the pool wall while keeping the feet flat on the floor.
- ▼ **Achilles Stretch:** Standing in neutral-facing position, exercisers bend the right knee and place the right foot forward, simultaneously extending the left toe straight behind the body until legs are about 12 to 16 inches (30-40 centimeters) apart; they press the left heel toward the floor while keeping the left leg straight (participants are now in a lunging position) (figure 6.25), hold for 8 to 12 counts, and return to neutral. Repeat this stretch for the right leg.
- ◀ **Push-back:** Beginning in neutral-facing position, exercisers flex the right knee to a 90-degree angle. Keeping the abdominals engaged and the low back straight, they press the knee back 6 to 8 inches (15-20 centimeters) (figure 6.26) and return to a 90-degree angle. Repeat 6 to 10 times, and then switch to the opposite leg.

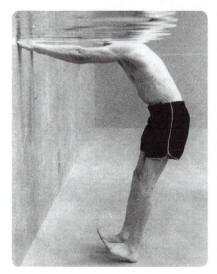

▶ **Figure 6.24** Rock-back.

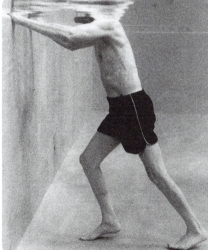

▶ **Figure 6.25** Achilles stretch.

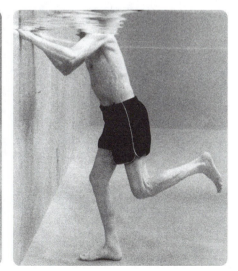

▶ **Figure 6.26** Push-back.

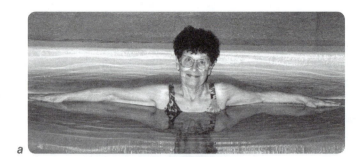

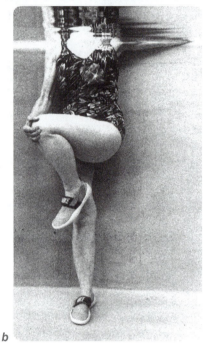

◀ **Cross-Knee:** With backs to the wall (figure 6.27a), exercisers lift the right knee to the chest (counts 1, 2), use the left hand to bring the knee across the front of the body to the left side (3, 4), and keep the shoulders square to the wall and hold (5, 6, 7, 8) (figure 6.27b), Then they bring the knee back to center (1, 2), open to the right side (3, 4), and hold (5, 6, 7, 8). Last they return to center (1, 2), bring the right foot back to the floor (3, 4), bend both knees (5, 6), and then straighten the knees (7, 8). They repeat the exercise on opposite side.

▼ **Side-Lift Turnout:** Beginning in neutral back position with the right leg slightly turned out to the right, exercisers slowly lift the right leg to the right side, keeping the right heel in contact with the pool wall (this should be a small lift) (figure 6.28); they hold and return to neutral. Then they repeat the movement to the left side with the left leg slightly turned out to the left.

▼ **Hamstring Stretch:** Beginning in neutral back position, exercisers bring the right knee to the chest and then, supporting the leg with the arms, extend the leg to the front, hold, flex the foot, hold, point the toe, hold, flex the knee back to the chest (figure 6.29), and return to neutral. Repeat the movement with the left leg.

▶ **Figure 6.27** (a) Neutral back wall position; (b) cross-knee lift.

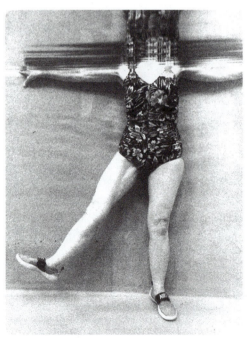

▶ **Figure 6.28** Side-lift turnout.

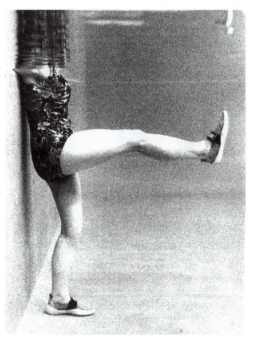

▶ **Figure 6.29** Hamstring stretch.

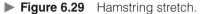

■ **Hip Circles:** Beginning in neutral back position, exercisers lift the right knee to the center, open it to the right side, draw clockwise circles by pulling the knee back and around to the center 6 to 8 times, return to neutral, and repeat on the left side.

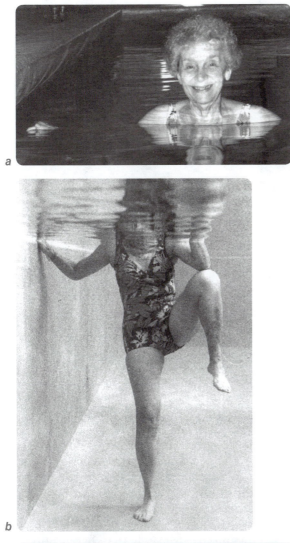

◀ **Knee Lift and Reach:** Standing in left-side neutral position (figure 6.30*a*), exercisers lift the left knee to the left elbow (figure 6.30*b*), bending at the waist to the left (counts 1, 2, 3, 4) (figure 6.30*c*), and then return the left foot to the floor while extending the left arm over the head and bending at the waist to the right (5, 6, 7, 8). They repeat the movement slowly 4 to 6 times and then switch to the opposite side.

▼ **Quad Stretch:** Beginning in left-side neutral, exercisers bring the left heel toward the buttock by flexing the left knee and then grasp the left ankle with the left hand to hold this stretch (figure 6.31). The left knee points straight down to the floor, and the right knee is slightly flexed. The abdominals are engaged to avoid hyperextending the back. Participants should avoid touching the left heel to the buttock because this hyperflexes the knee, placing it in a position vulnerable to injury. The stretch is repeated for the opposite side.

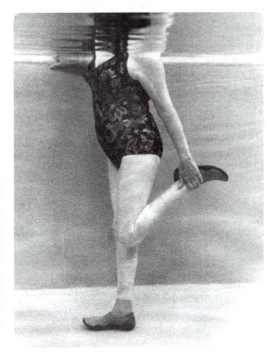

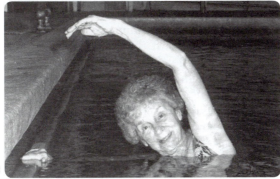

▶ **Figure 6.30** *(a)* Left-side neutral wall position; *(b)* knee lift; *(c)* reach.

▶ **Figure 6.31** Quad stretch.

All exercises done in the left-side neutral position should be repeated in the right-side neutral position, as illustrated in figure 6.32.

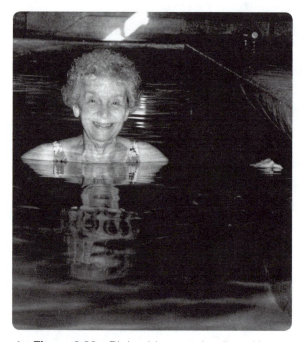

■ **Relaxation:** Allow some time (3-5 minutes) for complete relaxation at the end of the class. Use relaxing instrumental music and, if possible, dim the lights. Let students float in the water, do deep breathing, or perform their choice of relaxing activities.

▶ **Figure 6.32**   Right-side neutral wall position.

ARTHRITIS WATER EXERCISE

The arthritis water-exercise classes are designed to meet the needs of those who have arthritis, which significantly impairs the movement of one or more joints. These classes will also appeal to those with other physical limitations or those who prefer an exercise class that focuses on maintaining and improving range of motion and strength, with aerobic conditioning being a secondary goal. However, because water exercise may be one of the only forms of aerobic workout available to those with arthritis, an aerobic component should be included. The limitations in movement and the joint vulnerability posed by arthritis require special consideration to class format, water temperature, access needs, and specific exercise modifications. For example, the Arthritis Foundation has a list of requirements a program must meet before offering their Aquatics Program (Larkin, 2007). Extra attention to details will ensure that your program meets the special needs of this group.

Modifications to Class Format

The structure of an arthritis class is the same as a level 1 class. It will include 20 to 25 minutes of warm-up, range of motion, and strength work; approximately 15 minutes of aerobics; and 20 to 25 minutes of stretching and relaxation.

The exercises described in water exercise, levels 1 and 2, can also be used for arthritis water exercise; just keep in mind that you are dealing with people whose joints are significantly compromised by arthritis (see chapter 2 for information on arthritis dysfunction). For example, arm movements must be smooth and use the fullest possible range of motion. Program approximately 16 to 24 repetitions of low-intensity, low-impact aerobic movements and 12 to 16 repetitions of medium- to high-intensity aerobic movements with this group, and use transition movements for 16 to 24 counts between exercises. Use the high-intensity, high-impact exercises (such as jumping jacks) very sparingly, no more than 16 repetitions at a time. Avoid excessive flotation exercises and do not use exercises that require students to grip the side of the pool and support their body weight with their arms and shoulders.

Ask your participants for feedback: Is a particular exercise comfortable? Did they experience excessive soreness after the last class? (Exercise-induced soreness of the joints lasting 2 or more hours after exercise is a clear indication of overexertion.) The feedback you receive will help you help your participants gain the best results possible for the time they spend in class.

Water Temperature and Special Access Needs

Arthritis water exercise requires warmer water than a regular water-based exercise class. Many students with arthritis become uncomfortable during the warm-up and cool-down phases of class if the water temperature is below 87 degrees Fahrenheit (30 degrees Celsius). Water that is too cold can cause these students to experience discomfort and stiffness both during and after exercise. However, if the water is warmer than 90 degrees Fahrenheit (32 degrees Celsius), it is too hot to include an aerobic component. Even without the aerobic component, excessively hot water (92 degrees Fahrenheit [33 degrees Celsius] or above) is dangerous to exercise in or even be in for long periods. Those with high blood pressure and other heart-related conditions can become dangerously overheated, which increases their risk for cardiac problems. Even those without high blood pressure can experience dizziness, nausea, and fatigue when in water that is too hot. Continually monitor the pool temperature so you can adjust class format when necessary to ensure safety.

A class intended for those with arthritis must be held in a pool that provides easy access. Long stairways to the pool area can pose a barrier for those with severe arthritis in the knees and hips. A ladder that is the only access into the pool can present an insurmountable obstacle for those with severe arthritis of the shoulder or hands. Carefully evaluate your facility to determine whether you can offer a safe, accessible exercise class to this group.

Flotation and Wall Exercises

Plastic jugs can be difficult to grip or cause injury for participants who have severe arthritis in their hands. Therefore, noodles, water bells, or even adult-size water wings are necessary for flotation exercises. Regularly remind participants to only perform exercises through the pain-free range of motion.

Restrict flotation work to a maximum of 12 repetitions at a time to avoid excessive stress on the hands and shoulders. Take special care to alternate exercises that extend the arms to the sides with exercises in which the arms are bent and the devices are tucked under the armpits. (Keeping the arms extended to the sides for too long can cause shoulder soreness.) Have participants perform a maximum of two different exercises of 8 to 12 repetitions each in the extended-arm position before changing to an exercise that has the flotation devices tucked under the arms. Bicycling forward or backward is a good exercise to alternate with extended-arm exercises. Some participants will need to avoid being suspended in the water by their arms at all and instead can do modifications of the flotation exercises by keeping one foot on the floor or regularly touching both feet to the floor between exercises.

The same considerations apply to wall work. Participants with arthritis in their hands must not be expected to do wall work that requires gripping the pool gutter for long periods, so use those exercises very sparingly. Completely avoid exercises that require participants to grip the gutter and support the body weight with the hands and shoulders. When in doubt about the appropriateness of an exercise, weigh the potential benefits against potential risks and ask participants which exercises are comfortable and helpful.

For more specific guidelines and exercises, contact the YMCA program store at 800-747-0089 for information on the *Arthritis Foundation YMCA Aquatic Program Instructor's Manual*. This is an excellent resource that will give you many condition-specific exercises for this group.

WELLNESS WRAP-UP

Water exercise offers an excellent option for gentle to vigorous exercise with minimal stress on the muscles and joints. Programming in the water requires target heart rate modifications, special safety precautions and instructor training, and attention to details such as safe movement choices and appropriate water temperature and music. Regardless of class level, ensure that each class includes a warm-up, strength and range of motion work, aerobic conditioning, and cool-down and stretching. Control the level of aerobic intensity by alternating between very easy transition exercises and low-, moderate-, and high-intensity exercises.

Make time in class to integrate the whole-person wellness approach. The warm-up and cool-down phases in particular are the perfect times to encourage social interaction and create emotional connections among participants.

CHAPTER **7**

Developing and Promoting Your Program

Having the information you need to design safe, effective classes is only one part of the equation for creating a successful adult exercise program. Each venue is unique, and this chapter addresses developing and promoting programs in two environments: community-based environments, including community centers, senior centers, and fitness outlets; and senior-living environments, including age-restricted apartment buildings, continuous care retirement centers (CCRCs), and assisted-living and extended-care centers. This chapter discusses conducting a needs assessment, setting program goals, managing client relationships, and identifying appropriate facilities. It also outlines how to identify and reach potential clients and provides guidelines for effective promotional materials. Finally, it discusses challenges and opportunities unique to the senior-living industry and offers specific program approaches for this venue.

WORKING IN COMMUNITY-BASED ENVIRONMENTS

A needs assessment will help you determine interest in the community and develop your program goals. Consider the number of older adults in your community, other programs in existence, and the demand for adult exercise programming. Other important steps include finding a facility that will meet the needs of your program, devising strategies to promote your program, and motivating adults to begin—and continue—exercising. Careful attention to these details will ensure that the time and energy spent on developing your program are well directed.

Conducting a Community Needs Assessment and Setting Program Goals

Obtain age demographics for your area from the public library, chamber of commerce, and government agencies on aging. Contact the local senior centers, recreation centers, and fitness facilities to determine what exercise programs are currently being offered to mature adults. Take the time to evaluate any existing programs for your target population. Call as a potential participant to see what image the program staff project over the phone. The person who answers the telephone should be friendly and interested (but not patronizing) and should project a professional image, inquiring about your current level of physical activity and your goals for joining the program. If possible, visit the

program as either an observer or a participant. Talk to people in the program and listen to their praises and complaints. Then decide whether the needs of mature adults in your community are being met sufficiently by existing programs.

If you determine there is a need for your program, then you must become visible. Give talks or short workshops on exercise and health-related issues at the senior center, community club meetings, luncheons, or special events. This will advertise what you have to offer and allow you to gauge the level of interest in a new exercise program. And, of course, you must become an integral part of the network of senior services in your community. Carefully evaluate exactly how your program will fit into the senior services network, and then establish yourself as someone serious about providing a service to older adults.

Use the information gathered from your needs assessment to guide development of program goals. Write down program goals and objectives, such as increasing cardiovascular endurance, muscle strength and power, range of motion, balance, and coordination. Make sure that your program's efforts in these areas improve functional fitness (i.e., the level of fitness that people need to take care of personal needs, maintain independence, and engage in activities of choice). Two excellent resources are *Function Fitness for Older Adults* (Brill, 2004) and the *Senior Fitness Test Manual* (Rikli and Jones, 2001).

Set program goals for creating a positive social experience and improving self-esteem. Both of these elements play a significant role in motivating participants to continue attending classes. Improving well-being involves paying attention to multiple dimensions of health (see chapter 1), so your program should strive to improve as many of these dimensions as possible. In addition, consider the psychosocial elements that affect physical activity participation when creating programs and program messages (see chapter 3).

Interacting With Clients

The first phone call you receive from a potential client is an opportunity to start building a positive connection. Project professionalism in a friendly, interested manner, giving callers the specific information they ask for and asking important questions about their needs and goals. Ask about their current physical condition, recreational activities, whether they are now or have recently been involved in a regular exercise program, and what fitness and wellness goals they hope to achieve.

There are many reasons why people explore attending an exercise program. They may wish to improve their aerobic condition, strength, balance and coordination, or flexibility. Their goals may be less specific, like improving their appearance and health or improving their social life. Knowing what people hope to accomplish will help you determine how your program can best meet their needs.

When you have gathered the necessary information, explain how your program can help the caller accomplish her goals. If you offer a variety of classes, suggest those that will best meet her needs. This exchange of information should be conversational, not interrogative. Be prepared to talk with the client as long as necessary to obtain the needed information and learn a little something about this person, who may soon become part of your wellness "family." If you answer potential clients' phone calls with impatience or indifference, you can be sure they will not be motivated to take the next step—visiting your class.

The first time a potential client attends class, ensure a warm welcome by introducing him around. Generate a feeling of belonging among newcomers, just as you do for all participants in your program. Know your students' names and something specific about each of them, such as a special interest or talent. Make the time to visit with your students before and after classes, and take time during class for personal exchanges with and between participants. Generating a feeling of belonging to something special is a key to motivating people to begin and continue an exercise program. Refer to chapters 3 and 4 for strategies to facilitate this important component during class.

When people begin regularly attending class, encourage them to identify short- and long-term goals in each dimension of wellness, and provide an environment of support as participants strive to meet their goals. Time spent developing your program goals and encouraging whole-person health will ensure a well-rounded program and a feeling of belonging for all participants.

Identifying Appropriate Facilities

When choosing a facility for your exercise program, or when evaluating your own facility, consider its accessibility to physically restricted participants or those with hearing and visual impairment. Evaluate the facility's capacity for proper heating and cooling and its overall safety. If you are not already established at a particular facility, then, keeping these criteria in mind, explore local schools, churches, YMCAs and YWCAs, recreation centers, colleges or universities, senior centers, and fitness clubs. You may not find the perfect facility, but when making concessions, always remember—safety first: A program cannot continue if injuries are prevalent. A less than perfect facility should not prevent you from starting a program. It will simply mean that you need to develop your program with careful attention to the facility's limitations.

You may need to modify your program to fit your facility, for example, by using energetic chair aerobics rather than low-impact aerobics when the only exercise space available has an unsafe surface. When searching for the right movement space, do not disregard the option of providing a program without having a "base" facility. You may find it beneficial to take your program to the clients by scheduling sessions at several different places, such as senior centers, recreation centers, or senior-living communities. You can develop a successful program by providing classes on a regular basis at a variety of facilities.

Accessibility

Carefully gauge the facility's accessibility to people with a variety of physical restrictions, because lack of accessibility may limit your range of potential clients. Identify any obstacles that clients might encounter when coming to and leaving class. Evaluate where they will park, and watch for potential problem areas such as a long walk, difficult terrain, or excessive stairs. Consider seasonal changes, and remember that parking areas and walkways must have adequate snow removal, because snowy, slick surfaces can be obstacles to participation.

Scout out the route clients would follow getting to and from class, and identify any potential barriers to access. Some obstacles mentioned may not trouble participants who attend a low-impact aerobics class, but if you have a water aerobics or chair-exercise program geared toward those with physical limitations, you must identify and address any obstacle that might discourage or prevent their participation.

Suitability for People With Sensory Impairment

To determine whether a facility is appropriate for your clients, consider the suitability of its environment for people with hearing and visual impairments. The probability of having some degree of hearing or visual loss increases with age, so carefully consider whether your facility minimizes or compounds these issues. For example, in a pool area, you may be dealing with uncorrected hearing impairments, because most participants will not wear their hearing aids in the pool (just as some may not wear their glasses). An environment that is noisy because a variety of other activities are going on can be very uncomfortable for those with hearing loss and those with hearing aids. Competing background noise will make it impossible to hear directions, increasing participants' frustration and diminishing enjoyment. Those with hearing aids will experience amplification of all sounds, creating a jumble of competing noises. Most people will not return to a class that exposes them to such an uncomfortable experience. Make it a high priority to find a space as free as possible from background noise and competing activities.

Areas that are poorly lit and areas illuminated by direct sunlight or strong, reflected sunlight often trouble clients with diminished vision. Also pinpoint any place in your movement area that may pose a safety risk, such as a surprise step-off or a sudden change in floor texture. For a visually impaired participant, an unexpected change in floor texture could mean a fall. Check out parking lots and walkways when making your evaluation. Search out any surprise step-offs or level changes on the way to and from class. If classes are held at night, be sure the parking and walking areas are properly lighted.

Atmosphere

Determine whether your facility of choice has a welcoming and supportive atmosphere both inside and out. No one wants to feel out of place, so consider the type of music played, the primary clientele (bodybuilders and elite athletes or a broad mix), and the overall attitude of staff and members toward people over 50. Also consider the type of neighborhood environment clients must come through to access your classes at the time of day they will attend.

Finally, consider the location of the class within a facility. For example, scheduling a class in an area where participants could feel "on stage" (in the sense of being located where others are likely to stop and watch) can create an intimidating atmosphere, especially for beginners.

Heating and Cooling

Any exercise facility must have proper heating and cooling. This is an issue of not only comfort but also safety. It is dangerous for anyone to exercise in a room that is too hot. Overheated rooms are even more dangerous for anyone with high blood pressure and other conditions that can be complicated or aggravated by the heat. Aerobic exercise done in a hot room is especially dangerous and poses an unacceptable risk to participants. At the other extreme, a cold room makes it difficult to properly warm up

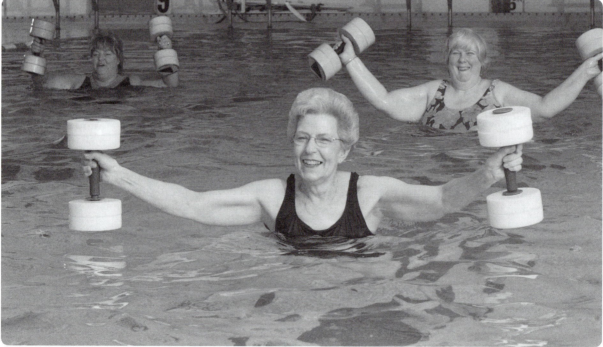

© Human Kinetics

Background noise can be a problem for aging participants, so try to eliminate competing activities in a pool area.

the muscles, making participants more susceptible to muscle pulls and strains. A cold room also promotes an undesirably rapid cool-down after aerobic exercise and makes an uncomfortable environment for stretching and relaxation.

Pool and Shower Areas

For any water-exercise program, you must evaluate the safety and accessibility of the pool, locker, and shower areas. If clients must negotiate stairs to access a pool area, people with functional limitations may not be able to access programs. That doesn't mean you can't have a program, but it does limit your potential client list to those able to climb stairs.

The locker room should be well lit, and the shower area should have a surface that minimizes slickness when wet. Evaluate the pool deck to determine whether slippery surfaces pose an unacceptable risk of falling. Footwear, such as aqua shoes, often can improve footing in areas with slippery spots, but do not allow clients to wear old tennis shoes, which may have worn soles and cause the wearer to slip on wet surfaces. Rubber matting (available through aquatics catalogs) can be a solution to slippery pool decks.

Evaluate the access into the pool itself. A stairway should have a solid railing to assist participants in entering and exiting the pool. A pool that has only ladder accessibility will make climbing in and out very difficult for those with upper-body limitations.

Exercise Surface

For land-based programs, the exercise surface is of utmost importance. A poor surface can contribute significantly to gradual deterioration of the joints and the possibility of acute injury. The best surface is a suspended wood floor like that in a gymnasium or dance studio. However, in the absence of such a feature, being aware of the potential risks can help you match the type of exercise you provide to the type of surface available.

The hardness of the exercise surface is a primary consideration. Performing aerobic exercise on very hard surfaces, such as concrete, is unsafe. The poured floors common in some multipurpose facilities and the thin exercise matting used on such floors can be too unforgiving on the knees, hips, and backs of participants. Be suspicious of carpeted floors, which are often only carpet over concrete. Even low-impact aerobics classes should not be performed on concrete or any other hard surface. If the only space available has an unsuitable surface (and you don't have access to cardiovascular equipment), you will be limited to chair-based aerobics.

The texture of the surface is also important. If the surface is slick and sticky or has numerous slick and sticky spots, it will increase your exercisers' risk of falling. Carpeting also poses some challenges to safety (even when laid over an acceptable surface), requiring you to adjust your movement combinations and patterns. Movement patterns will have to be very simple with minimal use of direction changes. Side-to-side movements, or any movement in which the foot drags across the floor, will pose a hazard. Such movements make it easy for a shoe to stick to or catch on the carpet, which can cause an ankle turn, trip, or fall. As always, weigh the benefits of each movement against the potential risks.

PROMOTING YOUR EXERCISE PROGRAM

Magazines and journals devoted to marketing are filled with information on how business is responding to the expanding older adult market. Marketing firms segment markets into age or generation and often view the older adult market through several market segments: 50- to 64-year-olds, 65- to 74-year-olds, 75- to 84-year-olds, and, the fastest-growing segment of all, the 85-plus category. As strategies evolve for marketing to senior consumers, ageless marketing is proving more effective than standard approaches (Snyder, 2002). Ageless marketing takes age out of the equation and addresses values, needs, and interests of consumers. Regardless of your approach, you should develop a network within the community, find your target clients, and create a consistent media message and delivery system.

Developing a Network

Marketing your program will depend largely on developing a cooperative relationship with other individuals and organizations that regularly provide services to your target market. One of the most beneficial steps you can take is to become an integral part of the senior services network in your community. This includes the senior center, area agencies on aging, county offices on aging, and a wide range of senior support services. If you are a visible and recognizable asset within this network, then your program will gain the credibility it deserves.

Make area physicians, physical therapists, orthopedic specialists, and chiropractors an important part of your network. Seek out their expertise and invite them to review your program. Ask their input on such things as the level of aerobic conditioning appropriate to clients with heart- and lung-related restrictions and the safety of your exercises for particular muscle and joint conditions. Most health professionals have very time-restricted schedules, so an effective method of opening the lines of communication may be to send a letter asking a specific question that can be answered briefly. You may find a health professional who has a special interest in older adult exercise and is willing to address your questions and concerns.

Strive to establish a relationship of trust and reliability. This will take time and attention to detail, but it will give a great deal in return. Adequately involving area health professionals will improve your program's safety and credibility. It may also increase participation through direct referrals from these health professionals. It is no secret that the right kind of exercise can improve many aspects of health; therefore, if area health professionals know you have a safe, effective program, they will gladly refer patients to your classes. While I directed the Bozeman, Montana, Young at Heart program, of the 200+ participants involved, approximately 40% were referred to the program by health care professionals.

If you are fortunate enough to live close to a college or university, include its health and fitness professionals in your network. They often can provide important, up-to-date information concerning specific exercise and other health-related topics and are generally more accessible than physicians.

Health and fitness professionals connected with colleges and universities may also offer opportunities for participation in research projects geared toward exercise for older adults.

Finding Clients

To develop a marketing strategy, you must first decide where to focus your marketing efforts. Consider where your target consumers do business, attend to their health needs, and congregate socially in your community. Once you have identified where your potential clients gather, then you can develop marketing materials appropriate for these locations.

Watch for businesses that provide special discounts or extra services to older adults. Look for clothing and grocery stores, gift and novelty shops, bookstores, restaurants, and barbers or hairstylists that your potential clients commonly patronize. For example, older, locally owned cafes may be favorites of long-time residents. Search for businesses that take special care to be friendly and accommodating to your target market, and focus your marketing efforts there.

Location is another factor to consider. Look for a grocery store within walking distance of senior housing or one that offers a delivery service. Locate shopping complexes that offer one-stop shopping. People without personal transportation may frequent stores where they can be dropped off and take care of all of their needs in one place.

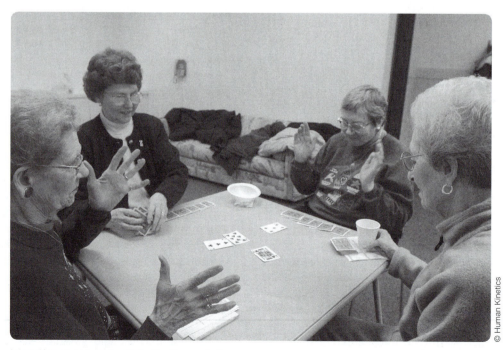

© Human Kinetics

Identify where potential clients socialize.

Consider where adults in your community are likely to go for health care. Look for a pharmacy with a convenient location or one that offers delivery service. If possible, identify community doctors who have a large clientele of older adults. These may include internists, family practice doctors, arthritis specialists, and doctors who have been in the community for many years. Most doctors' offices have a bulletin board where public notices can be posted. If you have a good relationship with area physicians, many will go a step further and place posters in examining rooms or hand out your materials to appropriate patients.

Finally, determine where people in your target market go to socialize. Senior centers, social clubs, city recreation centers, golf courses, bowling alleys, special community events, and night clubs with social dance music are some possibilities. Volunteer work is also an important social outlet. Identify community organizations whose specific focus is volunteer work, as well as organizations such as museums, hospitals, and churches that often large volunteer programs. When you determine where your potential clients go to enjoy themselves and engage with the community, you will have located places to focus your marketing efforts.

Using Media to Reach Clients

Develop strategies to reach potential clients through targeted newspaper, radio, and television ads. Older adults are the most loyal readers of newspapers, and newspapers are responding by significantly increasing their coverage of issues related to aging. Statistics reveal older television viewers' preference for news, sports, talk shows, and classic movies. The radio industry also notes that older listeners are significantly more likely to listen to all-news stations, news and talk formats, easy-listening programs, and nostalgia programs (Somerville, 2001).

Look for ways to use media outlets such as newspaper, radio, and television to reach your target consumers. Develop a mutually beneficial relationship with the local media—the key phrase here is "mutually beneficial"—by making yourself available to them and providing background information and assistance in your area of expertise whenever asked. Then, when you are ready to promote your program, you can use the ongoing media interest in aging issues to solicit local newspaper, television, and radio coverage. Sanner (2005) offers 10 tips for creating quality news releases: Always include contact information, date the news release, use a short and interesting headline, put the most important information first (who, what, when, where, why, how), keep releases short, write in the third person and keep it simple, use a "news" rather than "advertising" approach, limit expert quotes and keep them relevant, cite reliable resources for statistics, and carefully edit your release for proper style and writing.

■ **Newspaper:** Watch for national stories concerning research on the benefits of exercise for older adults. When the national news is focusing on these types of stories, contact your local papers to see whether they will run a story concerning this fitness research. Then place an advertisement about your exercise program to coincide with the article. If you have a program already established, this is the time to interest a local reporter in doing a feature on it as a follow-up or support article. Always inform your local newspaper of any special events your program is planning, and suggest the opportunity of a human interest story.

■ **Television:** The strategies suggested for local newspaper coverage are also appropriate for drawing local television attention. The time to interest a local station in doing a feature on your program is when national attention is focused on the benefits of exercise for older adults. Keep local stations informed of any special events your program is planning that may warrant human interest coverage on the local news. Area television stations may even be willing to do a live-broadcast segment, showcasing your exercise class in action. This can be great publicity and also a lot of fun for participants.

■ **Radio:** Local radio stations can be excellent avenues for publicizing your program. Select radio stations based on their focused market segment, and then plan your advertisements for when your target client is likely to tune in. Statistics show that older adults tend to tune into news programs on a regular basis. Although radio advertising representatives will speak of "drive time" (the time that people are likely to be in their cars with their radios on), these times coincide with the regular 8-to-5 workday, and many retired adults may stay off the road during peak traffic times. Work closely with a radio advertising representative to determine the peak listening times for your target market.

Paid advertisements are not the only way to take advantage of radio. Try providing health tips to be read on the air during public service announcement (PSA) breaks. Simple health information followed by "This tip is brought to you by (the name of the radio station) and (your program)" can do a great deal to publicize what you have to offer. Whether for an advertisement or a public service announcement,

Exercise Classes Are a Part of My Life

Helen, age 76, began exercising with the Young at Heart Program in Bozeman when it first began as a research project in 1995 determining the effect of exercise on older adults. Helen takes great pride in the fact that she has been enrolled in the program every session for all of these years. Asked what motivates her to keep coming to class, she says, "The exercise classes are really a part of my life. They just make me feel so good. If I miss class I really notice a difference and can't wait until I can get back to class." She adds, "My doctor is amazed at how flexible I am, and I know it is because of the water exercise classes.

"I really enjoy the other ladies. The social aspect makes coming to class more enjoyable because I know these people and enjoy visiting with them. I also enjoy meeting the new people who come to class and am happy when they find out how much better these classes can make you feel." Helen also uses exercise equipment at home, but she wouldn't give up her water aerobics classes for anything!

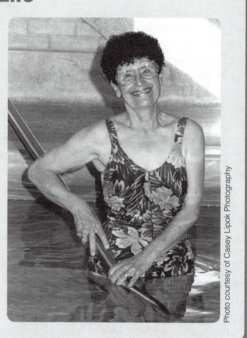

Photo courtesy of Casey Lipok Photography

consider using a catchy oldies tune as an introduction, but make sure that the dialogue is very clearly spoken without competition from background music. Close the announcement by repeating your contact information.

- **Online:** There is a huge push by industry and by health care and government agencies to encourage people to go to Web sites for information. According to a report by the Pew Foundation, Internet use stands at 54% among those ages 60 to 69 and ranges from 72% to 78% among baby boomers (Sipe, 2008). Create a Web site for your program that allows potential participants to look at a schedule of classes, read class descriptions, and see photos of participants in action. If you know how (or you know someone who does), consider posting links to short videos of classes. Make your contact information easy to find, and offer users the opportunity to ask questions through e-mail. Create a site that people will go to for information, even if you just provide a convenient list of links to reputable organizations with resources on wellness for adults.

Special Promotions

Special promotions, such as connecting your program with a special community event or even a data-gathering project, can generate interest in what you are offering. They give someone who has

been thinking about joining your classes a special incentive to take that first step. Special promotions can also be used to develop a core group of participants when you are starting a new program. It is critical that you have a well-planned program in place when you pursue a special promotion, because it will initiate the beginnings of a word-of-mouth network. When this network begins, it must be overwhelmingly positive if your program is going to benefit. Any event or project used only as a publicity stunt will do more harm than good if your program cannot deliver the expected results.

If you already have a core group of participants, consider staging an exercise demonstration at the senior center or a local shopping mall. You also can hold an open house for your program, allowing potential clients an opportunity to look at your facilities and observe or try out your classes for free. Look for opportunities such as Older Americans Month (May) to stage such events. Many national organizations, such as the President's Council on Physical Fitness and Sports, the U.S. Administration on Aging, the International Council on Active Aging, and the National Council on Aging, have posters and other media materials you can use for such events. You can also get involved in special events sponsored by local charities or fund-raisers devoted to community projects. Often, these events are centered on a walk-athon or other exercise-related activity, and having your exercise class participate as a group can bring visibility to your program.

It may also be beneficial to do a simple pretest–posttest data-gathering project with a group of clients to document the effects of exercise on specific components of fitness. Refer to the *Senior Fitness Test Manual* (Rikli and Jones, 2001) for a functional fitness test that is simple and does not require specialized equipment or excessive training. Advertising for participants for the project can bring in new clients who have considered joining your program and just need an extra incentive. This project also gives you the opportunity to send information updates to the local media that can generate further interest in your program.

On completion of the project, you will have data to use to promote your exercise program—information on improvement within the components of fitness and comments on personal progress and feelings of well-being gained through exercise. The positive results obtained by project participants will also generate positive word-of-mouth publicity that can bring many new participants to your program.

Program Materials

You probably will use a variety of posters, flyers, and pamphlets both to advertise your program and to communicate regularly with participants. If possible, consult a professional in marketing and graphics to help you develop the best promotional materials possible. These materials will influence your potential clients' first impressions of your program.

When creating promotional materials, take into account the needs of your target population. For example, the potential for having some degree of vision loss increases with age, so you must keep the design simple, uncluttered, and easy to read. Trying to squeeze too much information onto one item will diminish the visual clarity and discourage those with vision difficulties from trying to read your brochure. Use high-contrast colors, such as black print on white or yellow paper; even ivory-colored paper can lessen this contrast to a significant degree. Paper colors such as medium to dark blue, green, and red can make print very difficult to read. Even colored inks on white paper can be difficult to read, so use black ink for the text. The print itself should be slightly larger than average and consist mostly of simple block letters. Use flowery, scripted typefaces sparingly, because they can decrease ease of reading. Also avoid using numerous typefaces, which can cause a visually cluttered appearance.

Have an easily identifiable logo or graphic along with contact information to accompany all of your promotional materials. This gives potential clients something consistent to associate with your program, lends an image of permanence, and ensures that potential clients know how to contact you for more information.

Motivating Adults to Engage

The success of your marketing program will largely rely on how well you address issues that motivate your target consumer to action. You must provide motivation for people to begin your program and motivation for them to continue. Physical, social, and emotional factors have been proven to motivate people to begin and continue an exercise program. To achieve maximum response to your marketing efforts, address as many of these aspects as possible. Refer to chapter 3 for specific information on motivation and compliance.

Many adults who join an exercise program are motivated by a desire to improve their functional fitness and overall health and well-being. As discussed in previous chapters, functional fitness involves the physical capacities necessary to maintain an independent, active lifestyle and positive quality of life. These capacities include range of motion, strength and power, balance, coordination, and cardiovascular capacity and endurance. Therefore, your program must provide movement that matters in as many of these elements as possible.

You must educate potential clients on how exercise benefits them specifically. For example, leg strength, power, and flexibility allow people to engage in recreational activities like golf, travel, and mountain climbing. Becoming more physically fit translates to increased energy to engage in all activities of interest. When advertising your program, emphasize how it will specifically help participants maintain or improve independence and a positive quality of life.

Participants will be motivated to continue a program if they experience noticeable improvements in physical capacities and functional fitness or an overall feeling of improved health and well-being. If you offer a well-balanced program, participants should achieve noticeable results, so regularly assess and record improvements in cardiovascular function, strength, flexibility, overall mobility, and well-being. Solicit feedback from participants on how they feel about their progress. Help participants define individual short- and long-term goals and reward their successes with prizes and celebrations. Rewarding

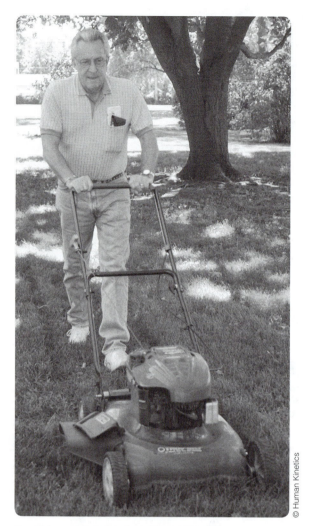

Exercise maintains functional fitness.

participation and goal attainment can provide the little extra motivation that people sometimes need to make exercise part of their lifestyle.

WORKING IN SENIOR-LIVING ENVIRONMENTS

This section addresses independent-living apartments with few or no services and communal-living arrangements with many services such as continuous care retirement communities (CCRCs), assisted-living communities, and extended-care centers. This section also identifies challenges posed by senior-living environments and provides ideas for developing and marketing programs.

Although senior-living environments have a built-in clientele and set location, you still have to actively market for participation in programs.

On average, only 20% to 30% of CCRC residents regularly participate in on-site exercise programs. In addition, of those not attending classes, only a small percentage report being regularly physically active in some other way. Clearly, having a built-in clientele does not ensure participation and a successful program.

Furthermore, don't assume that all exercise spaces will be optimal for your target group simply because they are located in a senior-living environment. Spaces are often used for multiple purposes, so assess the dedicated spaces for exercise programs in the same way you would assess a facility you are considering for a community-based program (see p. 141).

Carefully consider the group dynamics and wellness culture existing within the environment (i.e., attitudes toward exercise and other healthy lifestyle choices). Refer to chapter 3 to identify and remove hidden barriers to participation.

Independent-Living Apartments

Many communities have apartment buildings or developments that are age restricted (i.e., residents must be 55 or older). These age-restricted environments can range from low-income housing to upscale developments. Some buildings have an exercise area (often containing outdated equipment), but many have only multipurpose rooms. Many age-restricted apartments have no services or programs beyond what you would expect at any other apartment building. Some age-restricted developments have a clubhouse containing exercise equipment and spaces for meeting and socializing but seldom offer services such as meals and programs.

The biggest marketing advantage to age-restricted housing is that you can focus your efforts in one location. Interview residents and staff before starting your programs so you will understand the existing wellness culture in the building. Learn topics of interest to residents, and offer free health seminars. Visit with the people who attend these seminars and, if possible, visit residents who have expressed no interest in programs to help you understand some of the barriers to participation. Before starting your exercise program, distribute a questionnaire to residents asking about current levels of physical activity and attitudes about exercise and healthy lifestyle choices. Be sure to check with the on-site staff or the housing authority to ensure that you abide by rules for distributing materials and offering classes on site. Questionnaires should be very brief (one page), simple to fill out and

ACTIVITY SURVEY

Date:_____ Age:_____ Sex:_____ Code #:_____

For the purpose of this survey, *physical activity* is defined as going for a walk lasting 5 or more minutes, participating in exercise activities (individually or in a group), or participating in a hobby such as gardening, dancing, or bowling that requires sustained physical activity.

In the past 30 days, how many times *per week* have you been physically active? (circle one)

    0-1 times   2-3 times   4-5 times   6 or more times

How would you rate your overall personal health? (circle one)

    Poor   Fair   Good   Very good   Excellent

Please respond to the following statements by circling the response that best describes how you feel based on a scale of 1 to 5 with **1 being "strongly disagree"** and **5 being "strongly agree."**

	Strongly Disagree				Strongly Agree
1. Physical activity improves mental functioning.	1	2	3	4	5
2. I worry that physical activity could harm me.	1	2	3	4	5
3. Even though I'm older, I can become stronger.	1	2	3	4	5
4. I know how to be safe when physically active.	1	2	3	4	5
Regular physical activity can help me maintain or regain the ability to					
5. take a bath or shower.	1	2	3	4	5
6. get in and out of a chair.	1	2	3	4	5
7. go up and down stairs.	1	2	3	4	5
8. walk for 15 minutes at a casual pace.	1	2	3	4	5
9. reach overhead into cabinets or shelves.	1	2	3	4	5
10. I have a condition keeping me from physical activity.	1	2	3	4	5
Please specify _____					
11. I'm considering participating in an exercise program.	1	2	3	4	5
12. I believe that physical activity is important for health.	1	2	3	4	5

THANK YOU FOR PARTICIPATING IN MY SURVEY!

▶ **Figure 7.1** Sample activity survey.

From K. Van Norman, 2010, *Exercise and wellness for older adults,* 2nd ed. (Champaign, IL: Human Kinetics).

return, and confidential (no names necessary). This can provide tremendous insight into the culture of the environment. Refer to figure 7.1 for a sample physical activity survey.

Educate yourself on the group dynamics of the building and how they might enhance or detract from program participation. Maintain a friendly but professional approach; avoid commenting on or getting involved in any of the personal conflicts that might exist, but consider how you can minimize their impact on program growth. You may not be able to affect the dynamics, but it is important to understand them to give your program the best chance to flourish.

Continuous Care Retirement Communities

Continuous care retirement communities (CCRCs) usually offer three living situations in one complex: independent living, where residents live in apartments, town homes, or cottages and require no assistance with daily tasks; assisted living, where residents have their own room and bathroom and require daily assistance; and extended care, where residents have a room and bathroom and require daily assistance and rehabilitation or nursing services.

Many CCRCs have a fitness or wellness center with cardiovascular equipment (treadmills, stationary bikes, and seated steppers) and resistance training equipment. Some communities have a movement room to accommodate classes like low-impact aerobics, tai chi, dancing, and chair exercise. A CCRC might have a dining hall serving three meals a day in restaurant fashion, social areas, a salon or barber shop, in-house medical services, a wide range of physical activity classes, and a highly developed activities schedule. Although in most facilities all residents are welcome throughout the building and activities, there is usually a separate dining hall, separate multipurpose activity room, and separate activities for residents on the assisted-living and extended-care side of the building.

Assisted Living and Extended Care

Freestanding assisted-living communities provide services for people who are unable to live independently but do not require nursing care. Residents have their own room and bathroom (but usually no kitchen) or have their own room and share a bathroom. These communities usually have a mul-

tipurpose activity room and scheduled activities. Sometimes they have a dedicated fitness or wellness room with exercise equipment, but it is usually minimal. Chair exercise and rehabilitation services are the main forms of physical activity.

Most extended-care residents have significant mental or functional impairments. They have a shared room and bathroom or a private room and bathroom. There is usually a multipurpose activity room and a schedule of activities. In some cases there is limited cardiovascular or strength equipment, but it is primarily used for physical and occupational therapy. Chair exercise and rehabilitation exercises are the main forms of physical activity.

MEETING SENIOR-LIVING CHALLENGES AND OPPORTUNITIES

In any congregate-living environment (CCRCs, assisted living, or extended care) there are unique challenges to consider. The corporate or nonprofit culture is driven by the organization's mission, goals, and policies and by federal and state laws governing senior living. Extended-care facilities are very closely regulated, with frequent evaluations and surveys to ensure that residents' needs are being met. Assisted-living facilities have fewer regulations than extended-care facilities but more than independent-living situations. Sometimes these regulations make it difficult to implement new approaches to resident well-being. Take the time to understand these regulations and look for ways to frame wellness initiatives as an opportunity to meet specific survey requirements related to physical, social, and emotional well-being.

Staff dynamics are affected by the organization's culture, how well the mission and goals are articulated, and policies for hiring and training staff. Resident dynamics are affected by the organization's culture, staff dynamics, and the interpersonal relationships among people living in tight quarters. All of these factors contribute significantly to the overall culture of well-being in the senior-living community.

Organizational Culture

It is important to understand whether wellness programs in the senior-living community are considered part of the activity schedule (i.e., filling time slots) or whether there is an overall approach to resident well-being that strives to integrate wellness into all services and activities within the community. Part of the wellness approach is driven by the organization's policies and part is driven by the executive team. When you are the activity coordinator or leader at a senior-living facility, the relationship you develop with the executive team (e.g., chief executive office, chief financial officer, vice president of operations, and community director) will determine the support you receive for initiatives, which will dramatically affect your wellness programs. In addition, your relationship with the medical director will be important to the wellness program's success.

Look at programs from the perspective of the executive team, who are ultimately responsible for ensuring the long-term financial viability of the organization. Don't rely on the improvement of resident well-being as the sole rationale for program funding requests, because this is generally an expectation of all efforts within the community. Be able to clearly articulate how your programs specifically address the organization's identified mission, goals, and objectives.

Tie resident engagement in wellness programs to things like reducing costs, improving the ability to market the community to potential residents, improving functional status of residents, and improving resident satisfaction (thereby reducing turnover). Also learn to articulate how resident and staff wellness programs can improve employee recruitment, satisfaction, and retention. Employee salaries consume a large percentage of the budget, so finding and retaining good employees are chief concerns for the executive team. Jim Moore's book *Assisted Living Strategies for Changing Markets* and his Web site at www.m-d-s.com provide insight into the daily challenges faced by executives of senior-living businesses. Use this information to discover ways to frame your wellness programs as possible solutions to common challenges.

Staff and Resident Interactions

Work to engage all staff as active ambassadors for wellness. Talk to the directors of housekeeping, maintenance, medical services, and dining

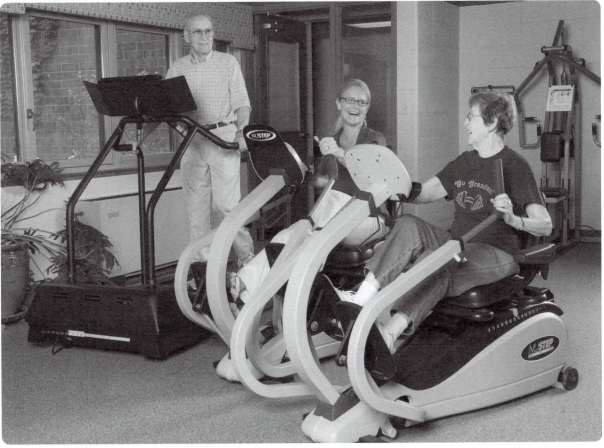

Residents and staff can share wellness opportunities.

© Human Kinetics

services to understand the responsibilities of each department. Make sure your exercise and wellness program goals are clearly articulated, and when scheduling activities consider how your programs may positively or negatively affect each area of responsibility. If your ongoing program or special event will inconvenience the staff or increase their work load, consider what can be done to mitigate that effect. Sometimes a simple conversation can prevent problems from developing, and acknowledging the extra effort made by other staff members to accommodate programs improves relations and communication.

Communicate frequently with the medical director to ensure she knows what exercise programs you are offering, what you do to promote participant safety, and how you coordinate efforts with the physical and occupational therapy staff. Look for ways to help the medical staff achieve their health management goals, and they will be more likely to encourage residents to participate in your programs. For example, work closely with physical and occupational therapists to help residents transition from therapeutic exercise into your exercise classes by discussing ways your program can help residents maintain gains they have made in therapy. Track the functional status of residents attending programs through simple functional assessments and share this information regularly with the medical staff. Many residents, especially those with significant health issues, rely very heavily on their health care providers' recommendations to guide physical activity behavior, so a positive relationship here can significantly affect program participation.

Every staff–resident interaction is an opportunity to either enhance or diminish wellness goals. Staff must be trained to consider how their actions (or inaction) can influence the attitudes and expectations surrounding wellness (see the sidebar). Make sure employees understand the key role they play every day in creating an environment of well-being. This requires a well-developed approach to staff training and ongoing education. Make sure new staff members learn about whole-person wellness the first time they enter the community. Advocate for wellness opportunities for staff as well as residents, and provide the human resources director with materials that articulate wellness goals and initiatives. Ensure that all department directors provide their new employees with simple, brief overviews of what makes the community a wellness environment. Materials should educate employees about what programs are available and request staff involvement in delivering wellness programs.

For example, in one CCRC a maintenance staff member (Ray) played the guitar and had an interest in teaching residents. The wellness coordinator negotiated with the community director to allow Ray to teach a half-hour guitar class to residents once a week during his normal workday without any negative impact on his pay. The food services director who worked in the same building loved history and volunteered to lead a history discussion each week. This approach increases visibility and credibility of programs but also offers a strategy to help address one of the biggest challenges in senior-living environments—recruiting and retaining quality staff. It actively fosters positive

RESIDENT–STAFF INTERACTION

A housekeeping staff member walks down the hall and observes a resident stopped in the hallway performing the functional task at a wellness station. The staff member

▶ smirks or chuckles and walks by (scenario 1);

▶ ignores the resident completely (scenario 2); or

▶ smiles, greets the resident by name, encourages his efforts, and perhaps even asks whether she can join him for a moment in the activity (scenario 3).

Scenario 1 demonstrates active discouragement, fostering embarrassment or shame to be "caught" exercising. Scenario 2 displays indifference and for a self-conscious person can act as passive discouragement of the wellness choice. Scenario 3 reinforces the resident's decision to engage. It creates a connection between staff and resident and actively supports an environment of well-being.

resident–staff interaction, improves morale, and sends a strong message that employees are valued as "whole people" who have much to offer beyond just filling a job. Seek support from your executive team for engaging staff in wellness activities by emphasizing how this approach can cost very little to implement but pay big dividends in improved staff recruitment, satisfaction, and retention.

Engaging staff both passively and actively in wellness initiatives is a crucial element to creating a community-wide wellness environment. Senior-living organizations wishing to market themselves as wellness communities often spend a great deal of time and money on wellness centers, programs, and equipment. However, failure to properly engage staff (at all levels and in all departments) will guarantee that wellness initiatives fall short of their potential return on investment. Visit www .kayvannorman.com for information on consulting services designed to help senior-living communities create and sustain environments of well-being.

Regardless of age or circumstances, every group will have its own unique dynamics. Be aware of resident dynamics without taking sides or getting involved. Usually there will be easily identifiable leaders who are involved in many programs and serve on advisory committees. Visit with leaders for insight on group dynamics, but avoid making judgments about other residents based only on the leaders' impressions. There may also be "natural" leaders who don't actively seek leadership roles but tend to be people whom others follow. To engage residents who are not currently involved in programs, seek out the natural leaders of this group to better understand the residents' perceived barriers to participation. Refer to chapter 3 for ideas on how to identify common barriers to engagement in wellness activities.

CRAFTING A CULTURE OF WELLNESS

Consider the influence each of the preceding elements has on the overall culture of the community, and seek opportunities to integrate whole-person

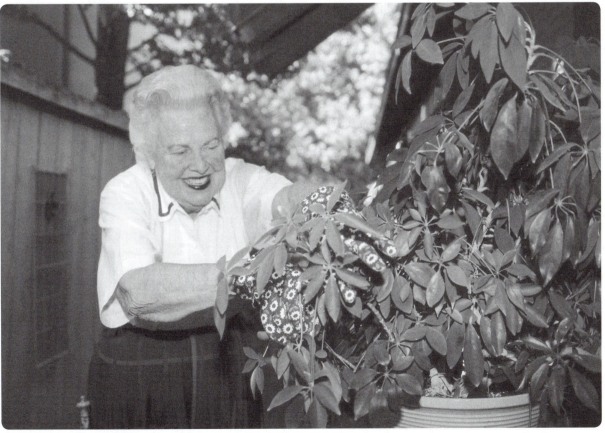

Gardening supports multiple dimensions of wellness.

Bill Crump/Brand X Pictures

wellness into the very fiber of daily life. There is a profound difference between using wellness programs to fill time slots in an activity schedule and fostering an environment of well-being for both residents and staff. Using the wellness approach doesn't mean that current programs need to be thrown out! Instead, the six dimensions of wellness act as a natural framework for all programming through the following:

■ Encompassing all aspects of body–mind–spirit wellness

■ Providing a means for evaluating existing program offerings and new program considerations

■ Providing continuity in wellness programs even amid staff turnover

■ Educating all staff and residents about objectives of programming

■ Helping both staff and residents view each other as whole people

■ Helping both residents and staff recognize potential areas of growth, regardless of challenges

■ Engaging residents and staff as active partners in their own well-being and enhancing their quality of life

■ Offering staff simple, specific strategies to work together to support resident well-being

■ Creating an expectation of well-being in the community and offering residents and staff strategies to support a wellness environment

Getting Started

An important step in creating a community-wide wellness environment is to carefully examine existing program offerings. Create a worksheet (see figure 7.2) for each dimension of wellness, and list program offerings under appropriate headings. Many programs can be listed under a couple of categories, but initially list them under the dimension reflecting the program's primary goal. For example, chair exercise would be listed under physical dimension programs but would also fit under the social dimension. This will provide a visual representation of which wellness dimensions are program rich and which ones need further development. Include medical wellness offerings as well as life-enhancement activities.

The column titled Ideas for Expansion encourages you to think about different approaches to programs within each of the dimensions. For example, the spiritual dimension is often only represented by religious services (of various denominations) and religious study. Consider adding programs that facilitate contemplation, reflection, and meditation to support personal growth in spirituality with or without a traditional religious focus. This will help address the complexities of the people making up your community of residents. Also facilitate the individual, self-directed involvement of residents. This can be achieved by simply providing residents with access to the necessary resources to try new things on their own. For example, in the physical dimension, make exercise props and self-directed brochures or videos available so people can choose to exercise on their own. The wellness stations illustrated in chapter 5 are an excellent example of self-

Dimension	Existing programs	Ideas for expansion
Physical	Exercise classes Walking clubs Health screenings Flu shots Gardening Nutrition programs	Activities of the week Wellness stations In-house TV channel movement breaks Walking meditation Massage therapy Physical therapy Tai chi stations Yoga stations Self-directed exercise resources (tapes, DVDs, brochures, resistance bands) Wii sports

▶ **Figure 7.2** Example of a partially completed wellness worksheet.

directed programs that address multiple dimensions of well-being. People can use the stations at their chosen days and times and at their preferred level of engagement. They may just look at the illustrations, read the positive affirmation statements, or stop to perform the functional exercise and pocket the takeaway item. Refer to chapter 5 (p. 81) for more information about using wellness stations as a unique wellness program.

Integrated Approach

Use the concepts behind Project MOVE (an acronym for motivation, opportunity, verification, and education) to create a balance between staff-led and self-directed activities, and encourage residents to become partners in well-being rather than merely customers of wellness offerings. *Motivation* refers to helping residents understand why a program is personally relevant to them; *opportunity* includes ongoing access to wellness opportunities at multiple levels, dimensions, and stages of change; *verification* refers to continual reinforcement of wellness con-cepts; and *education* involves a systematic approach to delivering information on wellness topics and opportunities. Refer to chapter 3, page 39, for a detailed description of the MOVE concept.

Table 7.1 illustrates how a common programming schedule from a senior-living community can be expanded into a more integrated approach using this concept. Self-directed opportunities for involvement help people take an active role in improving their quality of life. Creating a balance between staff-led and self-directed activities encourages residents to become partners in programming rather than just customers. Offering a variety of approaches within each dimension of wellness, at various levels of ability and stages of change, provides many points of entry into this lifestyle concept called wellness. Take advantage of opportunities to reach out both to current participants and to people who do not regularly participate in group activities.

This same integrated approach can be effective in initiatives for the broader community by engaging community outlets like churches, senior centers, senior service providers, and local businesses.

Table 7.1 Integrated Program Concepts

Primary dimension	Common existing programs	Ideas for expansion
Physical	Chair exercise	Home-based exercise brochures and equipment
	Other exercise classes	Activities of the week
	Flu shots	Wellness stations
	Health screenings	Physical activity breaks—before or after meals, after movies
	Gardening	Activity breaks that are broadcast on the internal TV station for multiple levels of functional ability
	Walking clubs	Walking circuits—inside and out, various distances
		Walking meditation
		Massage therapy
		Physical therapy
		Wii games
Social	Exercise classes	Active support for social interaction in exercise programs
	Bingo	Volunteer opportunities—mailings, phoning home-bound residents
	Walking group	Intergenerational activities with schools
	Trips to the mall	Internet access for communication with family and friends
	Club meetings	Coffee social with a specific topic of discussion (dealing with loss, investments, getting organized, humor and laughter)
	Church services and religious study	Opportunities to engage with the greater community—donate time and attention to local issue
		Ballroom dances, inviting community attendance and offering instruction by a local teacher
		Who's who—mixer games inviting interaction
		Wii games

(continued)

Table 7.1 *(continued)*

Primary dimension	Common existing programs	Ideas for expansion
Emotional	Movies Pet therapy Life-stories workshops Music programs	Positive affirmation training Wellness stations Thoughts for the day in exercise class, posted on bulletin boards Reinforcement on how increases in function increase self-efficacy Seminars on dealing with loss and grief Self-help techniques Walking meditation Nature interactions and outings Coffee social with a specific topic of discussion (dealing with loss, investments, getting organized, humor and laughter) Opportunity to contribute to the greater community (Retired Senior Volunteer Program [RSVP], knitting hats for infants at hospital) Intergenerational programs Massage therapy Aromatherapy Animal interaction Expression through training in the arts (music, dance, painting, sculpting)
Intellectual	Movies Guest lectures Group discussions Book clubs	Education on new technology: phones, DVDs, fax machines, computers Internet, e-mail, and Web cam training Education and discussion on positive psychology Education and discussion on aging and wellness Self-study manuals in subjects of interest Discussion of current events Brainstorming solutions for local issues Opportunity to teach hobby or skill Brain teasers as table tents or on bulletin boards Trivia teasers
Spiritual	Church services Religious study groups Religious TV services	Meditation and relaxation training and opportunities Wellness stations Walking meditations Volunteer opportunities Connections with nature Interaction with animals Discussions of life's meaning and purpose Designated and developed sites (indoor and out) for reflection and contemplation World religions seminars Spirituality book discussions Question-and-answer sessions with local religious leaders
Vocational	Club meetings Group discussions Gardening	Internet access for hobbies Volunteer opportunities Goal-setting workshops in all dimensions Discussions about focusing on possibilities rather than limitations Information about self-efficacy and self-motivation strategies Connection with the greater community through partnerships in giving Expression through training in the arts (music, dance, painting, sculpting) Wii games

Many local and state governments are looking for ways to increase physical activity and other healthy lifestyle opportunities for older adults, especially those who are considered to be at risk (e.g., homebound or physically frail people). Visit www.kayvannorman.com for information on how nonprofit organizations may be eligible to receive Project MOVE (described in chapter 5) for free.

WELLNESS WRAP-UP

Many wellness programs for adults are based at senior centers, community centers, and fitness clubs. Others are based in senior-living environments including age-restricted apartments, CCRCs, and assisted-living and extended-care centers. Community-based programs must find appropriate facilities, reach clients through promotions and marketing, and create an image that motivates potential clients to engage. Programs in senior-living communities have unique challenges and opportunities. They have easy access to a large group of adults but must still do a good job of marketing to engage residents in program offerings. Programs in all venues must provide an integrated approach that reaches residents at various levels of functional ability and stages of change.

The field of adult wellness is in its infancy. The baby boomers are just beginning to demonstrate their version of aging well, and people continue to write their own stories about what the last half of life should be like. Fitness clubs, senior centers, and community programs are trying to evolve along with this group. Senior-living environments may well see the biggest changes. Baby boomers are already influencing the industry by purchasing the senior-living "product" for parents or loved ones. But we have a long way to go before we can offer the optimal environment.

Creating six-dimensional models for programming and ensuring access to personally relevant opportunities constitute one layer of service for the senior population. Fostering positive attitudes and expectations for aging and health and supporting self-responsibility for health behaviors and outcomes are interconnected layers. All efforts are geared toward improving quality of life by engaging in activities with meaning and purpose. The real shift in this industry will occur when senior-living communities are developed around meaning and purpose. For example, development companies pour massive resources into developing the site plan, the function, and the appearance of the property inside and out. The marketing plan is designed almost simultaneously to draw potential residents with the location and the beauty of the development. Staffing, programming, and the social and emotional environment of the community are considered very important but are clearly secondary to the physical development of the property.

If we want to ensure quality of life and wellness environments, perhaps meaning and purpose should be the first things we consider when developing a project. What if new senior-living communities were built with a specific purpose in mind, that is, something that residents and staff would agree to work toward? For example, what if a senior-living project was developed around the purpose of growing organic produce for the greater community (e.g., schools, hospitals, senior centers, and food banks)? The grounds would be developed to house organic gardens and greenhouses, and the marketing plan would involve publicizing the meaning and purpose of the community. Of course, a community-wide culture of wellness would also be cultivated, but organic gardening would be an overarching purpose of the community. In the spirit of wellness, everyone could participate at their level of ability and self-selected level of involvement. Adaptive strategies would be used to facilitate participation by anyone who wanted to be involved, regardless of challenges. I can envision residents and staff of assisted-living communities and extended-care centers caring for animals in a petting zoo, inviting schoolchildren for regular visits, or partnering with a local animal shelter to care for and provide attention to the animals.

There are many worthwhile community programs that are understaffed and underfunded. If we take age out of the equation, then we can follow the lead of the disability movement. Young people with profound disabilities are given encouragement, strategies, and opportunities to live fully and contribute to their community, regardless of challenges. Frail older adults must be given the same encouragement, strategies, and opportunities.

I would love to see the day when marketing materials brag about how much organic produce is grown by community residents and provided to restaurants, schools, hospitals, and meal programs for the poor or highlight the number of children who visit the petting zoo, rather than focus on the beauty of the building and furnishings or how close the property is to health care providers. When we change our perceptions and expectations about aging and about the capabilities of adults with functional limitations, the possibilities will be endless and the potential outcomes exciting.

References

Administration on Aging, U.S. Department of Health and Human Services. (2005*). A profile of older Americans: 2005.* Washington, DC: U.S. Department of Health and Human Services,

Allen, J.V. (2005). Legal standards, risk management, and professional ethics. In C.J. Jones and D.J. Rose (Eds.), *Physical activity instruction of older adults* (pp. 351-363). Champaign, IL: Human Kinetics.

American College of Sports Medicine. (1991). Exercise prescription for cardiac patients. In *Guidelines for exercise testing and prescription* (4th ed., pp. 121-186). Philadelphia: Lea & Febiger.

Armstrong, S. et al. (2001). National blueprint: Increasing physical activity among adults age 50 and older [special supplement]. *Journal of Aging and Physical Activity* 9.

Bandura, A. (1997). *Self efficacy: The exercise and control.* New York: Freeman.

Barnes, D.E. (2004). *Action plan for diabetes: Your guide to controlling blood sugar.* Champaign, IL: Human Kinetics.

Benjamin, K., N.C. Edwards, and V.K. Bharti. (2005). Attitudinal, perceptual and normative beliefs influencing the exercise decisions of community-dwelling physically frail seniors. *Journal of Aging and Physical Activity* 13: 276-293.

Berger, B.G. (1989). The role of physical activity in the life quality of older adults. In W.W. Spirduso & H.M. Eckert (Eds.), *The academy papers: Physical activity and aging* (pp. 42-58). Champaign, IL: Human Kinetics.

Bloomfield, S.A., and S.S. Smith. (2003). Osteoporosis. In L.J. Durstine and G.E. Moore (Eds.), *ACSM's exercise management for persons with chronic diseases and disabilities.* Champaign, IL: Human Kinetics.

Boileau, R.A., E. McAuley, D. Demetriou, N.K. Devabhaktuni, G.L. Dykstsra, J. Katula, J. Nelson, A. Pascale, M. Pena, and H. Talbot. (1999). Aerobic exercise training and cardiorespiratory fitness in older adults: A randomized control trial. *Journal of Aging and Physical Activity* 7: 374-385.

Bradley, D.E., and C.F. Longino (2001). How older people think about images of aging in advertising and the media. *Generations, Journal of the American Society on Aging* 3:17-21.

Brill, P.A. (2004). *Functional fitness for older adults: Ready-to-use programs for improving quality of life.* Champaign, IL: Human Kinetics.

Brunner, F., A. Schmid, A. Sheikhzadeh, M. Nordin, J. Yoon, and V. Frankel. (2007). Effects of aging on type II muscle fibers: A systematic review of the literature. *Journal of Aging and Physical Activity* 15: 336-348.

Bryant, C.X., and Green, D.J. (Eds. 2005). *Exercise for older adults: ACE guide for fitness professionals.* San Diego: American Council on Exercise.

Buettner, D. (2005). The secrets of long life. *National Geographic*, November 2005.21-30.

Bylina, M.M., T. Hu, T.J. Conway, J. Perrin, J.L.E. Houser, J. Hurst, and C.C. Cox. (2006). Comparison of exercise attitudes and behaviors of urban older adults with AARP's national sample results. *Journal of Aging and Physical Activity* 14: 41-58.

Centers for Disease Control and Prevention and the Merck Company Foundation. (2007). *The state of aging and health in America.* Whitehouse Station, NJ: Merck Company Foundation.

Cheung, C., J. Wyman, C. Gross, J. Peters, M. Findorff, and H. Stock. (2006). Exercise behavior in older adults: A test of the transtheoretical model. *Journal of Aging and Physical Activity* 15: 103-118.

Chodzko-Zajko, W.J. (2005). Physiology of aging and exercise. In C.X. Bryant and D.J. Green (Eds.), *Exercise for older adults: ACE guide for fitness professionals* (pp. 2-23). San Diego: American Council on Exercise.

Christensen, C.L., V.G. Payne, E.H. Wughalter, and H.H. Yan. (2003). Physical activity, physiological, and psychomotor performance: A study of variously active older adult men. *Research Quarterly for Exercise and Sport* 74: 136-142.

Clark, D.O., T.E. Stump, S.L. Hui, and F.D. Wolinsky. (1998). Predictors of mobility and basic ADL difficulty among adults aged 70 years and older. *Journal of Aging and Health* 10(4): 422-440.

Coalman, M. (2007). Positive psychology: A new way to support wellness in older adults? *Journal on Active Aging* 6(4): 51-55.

Cohen, G.D. (2005). *The mature mind. The positive power of the aging brain.* New York: Basic Books.

Cohen-Mansfield, J., Marx, M.S., Guralnik, J.M (2003). Motivators and barriers to exercise in an older community-dwelling population. *Journal of Aging and Physical Activity* 11: 242-253.

Cousins, S.O. (1997). Elderly tomboys? Sources of self-efficacy for physical activity in late life. *Journal of Aging and Physical Activity* 5(3): 229-243.

Dishman, R.K. (1994). Motivating older adults to exercise. *Southern Medical Journal* 87(5): 79-82.

Durstine, L.J., and Moore, G.E. (Eds.) (2003). *ACSM's exercise management for persons with chronic diseases and disabilities.* Champaign, IL: Human Kinetics.

Elkowitz, E.B., and D. Elkowitz. (1986). Adding life to later years through exercise. *Exercise in the Elderly* 80(3): 92-94.

Ferebee-Eckman, T. (2008). Dance for older adults: A fun approach to exercise. *Journal on Active Aging* 7(4): 50-57.

Fiatarone, M. (1994). Exercise training and nutritional supplementation for physical frailty in very elderly people. *New England Journal of Medicine* 330:1769-1775.

Fielding, R.A., N.K. LeBrassuer, A. Cuoco, J. Bean, K. Mizer, and M.A. Fiatarone-Singh. (2002). High velocity resistance training increases skeletal muscle peak power in older women. *Journal of the American Geriatric Society* 4: 655-662.

Foldvari, M., M. Clark, L.C. Laviolette, M.A. Bernstein, D. Kaliton, C. Castaneda, C.T. Pu, J.M. Hausdorff, R.A. Fielding, and M.A. Singh. (2000). Association of muscle power with functional status in community-dwelling elderly women. *Journal of Gerontology: A. Biological Science Medical Science* 55(4): M192-199.

Goldberg, A.P., and Hagberg, J.M. (1990). Physical exercise in the elderly. In E. Schneider and J.W. Rowe (Eds.), *Handbook of the biology of aging* (pp. 407-423). San Diego: Academic Press.

Gordon, N.F. (2003). Hypertension. In L.J. Durstine, and G.E. Moore (Eds.), *ACSM's exercise management for persons with chronic diseases and disabilities* (pp. 76-80). Champaign, IL: Human Kinetics.

Gordon, N.F. (1993). *Diabetes: Your complete exercise guide.* Champaign, IL: Human Kinetics

Hagberg, J.M. (1988). Effect of exercise and training on older men and women with essential hypertension. In W.W. Spirduso and H.M. Ecker (Eds.), *The academy papers: Physical activity and aging (pp. 186-181)*. Champaign, IL: Human Kinetics.

Hagberg, J.M., J. Park, and M.D. Brown. (2000). The role of exercise training in the treatment of hypertension. *Sports Medicine* 30: 193-206.

Hall, C.D., A.L. Smith, and S.W. Keele, and W. Steven. (2001). The impact of aerobic activity on cognitive function in older adults: A new synthesis based on the concept of executive control. *European Journal of Cognitive Psychology* 13: 279-300.

Hawkins, S.A., R.A. Wiswell, and E.T. Schroeder. (2002). The relationship between bone adaptations to resistance exercise and reproductive hormone levels. *Journal of Aging and Physical Activity* 10: 64-75.

Hazell, T., K. Kenno, and J. Jakobi. (2003) Training for muscle power in older adults: Effects on functional abilities. *Canadian Journal of Applied Physiology* April;28(2):178-89.

Hazell, T., K. Kenno, and J. Jakobi. (2007). Functional benefit of power training for older adults. *Journal of Aging and Physical Activity* 15: 349-359.

Holland, G.J., K. Tanaka, R. Shigematsu, and M. Nakagaici. (2002). Flexibility and physical functions of older adults: A review. *Journal of Aging and Physical Activity* 10: 169-206.

Hornsby, G.W. and Albright, A.L. (2003). Diabetes. In L.J. Durstine and G.E. Moore (Eds.), *ACSM's exercise management for persons with chronic diseases and disabilities* (pp. 133-141). Champaign, IL: Human Kinetics.

Jones, C.J. and J. Clark (1998). National standards for preparing senior fitness instructors. *Journal of Aging and Physical Activity* 6: 207-221.

Jones, C.J., and R.E. Rikli. (1994). The revolution in aging: Implications for curriculum development and professional preparation in physical education. *Journal of Aging and Physical Activity* 2: 261-272.

Jones, C.J., and Rose, D.J. (2005). *Physical activity instruction of older adults.* Champaign, IL: Human Kinetics.

Kinsella, K., and D.R. Phillips (2005). Global aging: The challenge of success. *Population Bulletin. A Publication of the Population Reference Bureau* 60(1).

Kreighbaum, E. (1987). Anatomy and kinesiology. In N. Van Gelder (Ed.), *Aerobic dance exercise instructor manual* (pp. 35-88). San Diego: International Dance-Exercise Association (IDEA) Foundation.

Krueger, B. (2001). How aging is covered in the print media. *Generation: Journal of the American Society on Aging* 3: 10-12.

Larkin, M. (2007). Arthritis: innovative, evidence-based programs get results. *Journal on Active Aging* 6(4): 40-47.

Lees, F.D., P.G. Clark, C.R. Nigg, and P. Newman. (2005). Barriers to exercise behavior among older adults: A focus-group study. *Journal of Aging and Physical Activity* 13: 23-33.

Lucidi, F., C. Grano, C. Barbaranelli, and C. Violani. (2006). Social-cognitive determinants of physical activity attendance in older adults. *Journal of Aging and Physical Activity* 13: 344-359.

MacRae, H. (2005). Cardiovascular and pulmonary function. In W.W. Spirduso, K.L. Francis, and G.M. Priscilla (Eds.), *Physical dimensions of aging* (pp. 87-106). Champaign, IL: Human Kinetics.

MacRae, P.G. (1986). The effects of physical activity on the physiological and psychological health of the older adult. In D.A. Peterson, J.E. Thornton, and J.E. Birren (Eds.), *Education and aging* (pp.205-230). Englewood Cliffs, NJ: Prentice Hall.

Masoro, E.J. (1999). *Challenges of biological aging.* New York: Springer.

Maynard, K. (2005). *No excuses. The true story of a congenital amputee who became a champion in wrestling and in life.* Washington, DC: Regnery.

Minor, M.A., and Kay, D.R. (2003). Arthritis. In L.J. Durstine and G.E. Moore (Eds.), *ACSM's exercise management for persons with chronic diseases and disabilities* (pp. 210-216). Champaign, IL: Human Kinetics.

Miszko, T.A., M.E. Cress, J.M. Slade, C.J. Covey, S.K. Agrawal, and C.E. Doerr. (2003). Effect of strength and power training on physical function in community-dwelling older adults. *Journal of Gerontology: Medical Sciences* 58(2): 171-175.

Montague, J., and K. Van Norman. (1998). The multi-stations wellness model. *Assisted Living Success*, August.

Moore, J. (2002). *Assisted living strategies for changing markets.* Fort Worth, TX: Westridge Publishing.

Morgenthal, A.P., and R.J. Shephard. (2005). *Physiological aspects of aging.* In C.J. Jones and D.J. Rose (Eds.), *Physical activity instruction of older adults* (pp. 38-51). Champaign, IL: Human Kinetics.

National Institute on Aging. (1990). *Physical frailty: A reducible barrier to independence for older Americans.*

Nelson ME, Fiatarone MA, Morganti CM, Trice I, Greenberg RA, Evans WJ (1994). Effects of high intensity strength training on multiple risk factors for osteoporotic fractures: A random controlled trial. *Journal of the American Medical Association* 272(24): 1909-1914.

O'Brien Cousins, S. (2001). Thinking out loud: What older adults say about triggers for physical activity. *Journal of Aging and Physical Activity* 9:347-363.

Pappas-Gaines, M.B. (1993). *Fantastic water workouts. Low impact water exercises for health and fitness.* Champaign, IL: Human Kinetics.

Prochaska, J.O., and Marcus, B.H. (1994). The trans-theoretical model: Application to exercise. In R.K. Dishman (Ed.), *Advances in exercise adherence* (pp.161-179). Champaign, IL: Human Kinetics.

Rasinaho, M., M. Hirvensalo, R. Leinonen, T. Lintunen, and T. Rantanen. (2007). Motives for the barriers to physical activity among older adults with mobility limitations. *Journal of Aging and Physical Activity* 15: 90-102.

Ray, O. (2004). How the mind hurts and heals the body. *American Psychologist* 59(1): 29-40.

Rikli, R.E., and Jones, C.J. (2001). *Senior fitness test manual.* Champaign, IL: Human Kinetics.

Rimmer, J.H. (2005a). Common health challenges faced by older adults. In C.X. Bryant and D.J. Green (Eds.), *Exercise for older adult: ACE guide for fitness professionals* (pp. 77-96). San Diego: American Council on Exercise.

Rimmer, J.H. (2005b). Exercise considerations for medical conditions. In C.J. Jones and D.J. Rose (Eds.), *Physical activity instruction of older adults* (pp. 335-348). Champaign, IL: Human Kinetics.

Rose, D.J. (2003). *FallProof: A comprehensive balance and mobility training program.* Champaign, IL: Human Kinetics.

Sanders, M. (2008). Cultivating a water exercise program using an evaluation approach. *Journal on Active Aging* 7(1): 57-64.

Sanner, B. (2005). Effective news releases. *Journal on Active Aging* 4: 2

Semerjian, T., and D. Stephens. (2007). Comparison style, physical self-perceptions, and fitness among older women. *Journal of Aging and Physical Activity* 15: 219-235.

Shephard, R.J. (1999). Determinates of exercise in people aged 65 years and older. In R.K. Dishman (Ed.), *Advances in exercise adherence* (pp. 343-360). Champaign, IL: Human Kinetics.

Sipe, C. (2008). On-line learning for the 50-plus adult. *Journal on Active Aging* 7(1): 34-40.

Smith, E.L., and C. Gilligan. (1989a). Biological aging and the benefits of physical activity. In D.K. Leslie (Ed.), *Mature stuff: Physical activity for the older adult* (pp. 45-60). Reston, VA: American Alliance for Health, Physical Education, Recreation and Dance.

Smith, E.L., and C. Gilligan. (1989b). Osteoporosis, bone mineral, and exercise. In W.W. Spirduso and H.M. Eckert (Eds.), *The academy papers: Physical activity and aging* (pp. 106-113). Champaign, IL: Human Kinetics.

Snyder, R. (2002). Ageism in advertising. *Journal on Active Aging* 1(5): 12-14.

Somerville, R. (2001). Demographic research on newspaper readership. *Generations: Journal of the American Society on Aging* XXV(1): 24-30.

Sova, R. (2005). Aquatic training. In C.J. Jones and D.J. Rose (Eds.), *Physical activity instruction of older adults* (pp. 335-348). Champaign, IL: Human Kinetics.

Spirduso, W.W., K.L. Francis, and P.G. MacRae. (2005). *Physical dimensions of aging.* Champaign, IL: Human Kinetics

Stamford, B.A. (1988). Exercise and the elderly. *Exercise and Sport Sciences Review* 16: 341.

Stelmach, G.E., and N.L. Goggin. (1989). Psychomotor decline with age. In W.W. Spirduso and H.M. Eckert (Eds.), *The academy papers: Physical activity and aging* (pp. 6-18). Champaign, IL: Human Kinetics.

Umstattd, M.R., and J. HallamJ. (2007). Older adults' exercise behavior: Roles of selected constructs of social-cognitive theory, *Journal of Aging and Physical Activity* 15: 206-218.

Van Norman, K. (2004). Increasing physical activity participation among 50+ adults: A new approach. *Journal on Active Aging* 3: 32-38.

Wilmore, J.H. (1988). Exercise-drug interactions in the older adult. In W.W. Spirduso and H.M. Eckert (Eds.), *The academy papers: Physical activity and aging* (pp. 194-199). Champaign, IL: Human Kinetics.

Wise, J.B., & Trunnell, E.P. (2001). The influence of sources of self-efficacy upon efficacy strength. *Journal of Sport and Exercise Psychology* 23: 268-280.

World Health Organization. (2005). *Preventing chronic diseases: A vital investment.* http://whqlibdoc.who.int/publications/2005/9241593598_eng.pdf.

Index

Note: The italicized *f* and *t* following page numbers refer to figures and tables, respectively.

About the Author

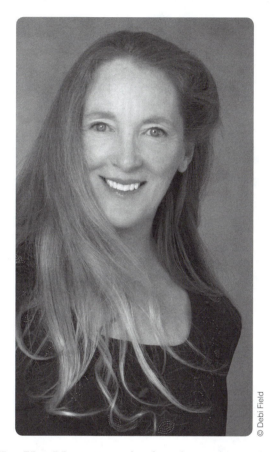
© Debi Field

Kay Van Norman is the founder and president of Brilliant Aging, a consulting firm specializing in older adult wellness. With a master's degree in physical education and health, she taught for the department of health and human development at Montana State University from 1981 to 1999 and directed MSU's Young at Heart exercise program for older adults from 1989 to 1998. She also served as the 1995-1997 national chair of the Council on Aging and Adult Development within the American Alliance for Health, Physical Education, Recreation and Dance. From 1999 to 2002, Ms. Van Norman served as director of the Keiser Institute on Aging, an international effort to bridge the gap between research and practice in the fields of gerontology, senior housing, fitness, and older adult wellness.

A leading authority in older adult wellness, Ms. Van Norman has authored numerous book chapters and more than 20 national and international journal articles on the subject. She authored a 2006 issue brief for the National Council on Aging examining the role of ageism on health behaviors. As a consultant, Ms. Van Norman designs comprehensive wellness programs for senior housing, creates wellness resources, conducts staff training, and regularly speaks at national and international conferences.

Ms. Van Norman received the 1998 Rosabel Koss Honor Award for her service to the profession of older adult health and a 2003 Best Practices Award from the National Council on Aging for her innovative products meeting the needs of older adults. She currently serves as a delegate for the Health Promotion Institute of the National Council on Aging and serves on the boards of the International Council on Active Aging and the American Senior Fitness Association.

The following services and products are available through Brilliant Aging:

- Keynote and breakout session speeches
- Wellness program design and development
    - Staff training
    - Resident seminars
- Community and statewide wellness initiatives
    - Reaching at-risk older adults
    - Leveraging program dollars with matching grants
    - Evidence-based programs
- Resources
    - Whole-person wellness stations
    - Educational curriculums
    - Project MOVE
    - Activities of the week series
    - Videos and DVDs: low-impact aerobics, chair exercise
- Brilliant Aging membership services
    - Downloadable resources
    - Interactive Web-based community

Visit www.kayvannorman.com or contact Kay at kayvn@kayvannorman.com.